Pay Close
to That Man Behind the
Curtain

and other stories

or

*What You Don't Know About Your
Medical Care Can Hurt You*

Dr. Bob Sinsheimer

First Edition Published 8/13/2022.
Second Edition Published 10/19/2022
(2nd edition incorporates corrections of diction and punctuation and adds an index. Also brings lines closer together)

Pay Close Attention to That Man Behind the Curtain

and other stories

or

What You Don't Know About Your Medical Care Can Hurt You.

Notes about people in this book: I am not attempting to attack any doctors, companies, or other individuals in this book. I am critical of the *behaviors* of some people. Those behaviors are common enough. They are not unique to the people in these stories. I reveal these behaviors not to attack anyone. My purpose is to help patients protect themselves. I think it's safe to say there are no bad doctors in this book. Every example of bad behavior described was by a physician who I am confident did MANY MORE good things than bad in their careers. The identities of the doctors and the patients have all been disguised except for a few doctors who are named to give them the praise they are due.

ABOUT THE BOOK:

This is a book for patients who value our healthcare "system," but who don't trust it and who want to avoid the hazards that may result from not realizing that they didn't understand it. In a nutshell, it is for people who want to be "smarter patients." Also, this book is for friends and families of any patient who may need this help. This is a book for people who can understand that one way to avoid those hazards is by learning about how doctors think, how they make errors, and how they are influenced by bias. These topics may appeal to people who would never dream of picking up a book about healthcare but who are curious about it and like to learn through stories that teach. This is book for people who would prefer to read three or four pages to get to the point rather than wade through an entire book on a single subject. To better communicate these ideas, the text is filled with short sentences and brief chapters. Many lessons learned over the past 50 years are disclosed on these pages. This book is also for patients who would like to share more in decisions made about their medical care if only their doctors would explain more. This book might encourage some patients who might need a little push to assert themselves when their doctor does not answer their questions. Finally, this is a book for people who want to know more than a little something about the author whose opinions they are reading.

About the author...

In addition to the practice of Family Medicine for 42 years, for seven years Dr. Bob Sinsheimer served as the chief physician at two community hospitals. In that role, he was responsible for investigating and learning from the errors of hundreds of doctors. This experience gave him a perspective very different from most physicians. He decided the best way to improve medical care was to study doctors' errors. In that way, lessons could be shared confidentially with the doctors and then with a wider number of doctors who treated the same conditions. It's now time to share many of those lessons with patients.

Comments by readers...

"Bob is a natural storyteller, and his career has presented him with many stories to tell. The reader hardly recognizes that serious, important points are being made in a most disarming way. His writing style appreciates the value of brevity: short preface, short chapters, short sentences. I read through these pages and wanted to keep going!"
Ray Ollwerther, retired managing editor of the Princeton Alumni Weekly.

"In the world of medicine, what you don't know might just kill you. Dr. Sinsheimer has given us the understanding we need to navigate this world. He speaks to us like the wise and caring family doctor we all wish we had today."
Jim Koch, founder and brewer of Sam Adams Beer and Chairman of Boston Beer Company.

"In his book, "Pay Close Attention to That Man Behind the Curtain and other stories or What You Don't Know About Your Medical Care Can Hurt You," Dr. Bob Sinsheimer MD takes the reader on an unforgettable journey of incredible stories. Like Aladdin's magical carpet, the author zig zags thru a variety of topics and interests, creatively and humorously, leaving no room for boredom. He shares with the reader his firsthand knowledge from his 42 years of family medical practice and medical leadership, through lessons learned from patients and other physicians. Dr. Sinsheimer, a Princeton All-American swimmer, lets the reader in on his innovative theory of aerodynamic swimming, as well as his genuine interest in cultures, people, and reflections on the concepts of heaven and hell. The author warns readers not to be passive patients, but to take an active role in understanding their care. As you read every story, not only do you get to see what's "Behind the Curtain" but you also meet the man pulling the curtain open for you, an articulate, creative, out-of-the box thinker, both unconventional and hilariously funny.
Fatimah Deffaa, Founder of the first women's bank in Saudi Arabia for Citibank Riyadh.

"My first impression is not of the essays, but of you. You appear to be the epitome of a doctor. You sound dedicated and compassionate and are obviously a good listener. I found each chapter to be well explained, well written, informative or amusing. I feel like I got a lot of good advice and was also entertained."
Jan Krawczyk.

"As a 30 something teacher is in good health, I didn't know what to expect from a nonfiction book written for patients. I was drawn into the engaging stories from Dr. Sinsheimer's career and I learned a thing or two along the way."
Erin Jahnke, Elementary School Teacher.

"Telling medical stories that both inform and amuse is hard to do but Dr. Sinsheimer makes it seem easy. This book is a light, enjoyable, and valuable read for any patient."
Ronald J. Liss, president and founder of the American Patient Rights Association.

More...from the author...

I decided the shortest description of what I did in practice was "Help Patients Make Smarter Decisions". I continue that quest with this book.

I realized that few reasonable persons would actually choose to read about topics which on the surface sound uninteresting despite being important: shared medical decision making, informed consent, and patient safety (meaning freedom from being harmed by medical errors). People become very interested in their rights when they face losing them. But in the case of the right of patients to be informed so they can protect themselves, here are rights which have been granted by society but which are underutilized. In 42 years of practice after medical school, I saw too many cases where the patient would have done better had they had been better informed. I decided to describe what I had learned through short, humorous anecdotes, jokes, and true stories from my career. Some are disturbing, others are inspiring."

Through stories, brief discussions, and quirky humor, I try to show the reader about how the pressure to see patients faster affects how doctors reason, and can result in errors. I explore physician ethics, physician bias, and how the practice of medicine includes assumptions that may someday be proven wrong. I explain how conventional practices often continue to be used after newer ones have been shown to work better. I try to make understandable some difficult but important topics such as how early detection by screening tests can falsely appear to be improving cancer survival statistics. I discuss how to ask questions about proposed tests or treatments which sometimes are known to help only a small percentage of patients or may harm more patients than patients realize.

Some of the more biographical stories in the book may relate to the medical themes in the book (or not): How I participated in a victimless crime that lead to the creation of an award given at Princeton for the past 50 years. A harrowing journey in a small airplane. A chance decision at age nine that affected the rest of my life. A lesson I learned at age ten after challenging my doctor's treatment for a cough.

Among the themes, topics, and stories found in the book:

Can you trust a doctor who is always on time?
Medical truths are not black or white.
Trust a doctor who makes errors and learns from them.
Beware the doctor impaired by avarice.
Be careful what you sign.

What to do about those monkeys in your mother's trees.
Safe and effective is not necessarily "cost effective" to the FDA.
How a bidet might save you thousands of dollars.
Doing nothing can be the best option.
We have our own Witch Doctors.
Eating one saltine at a time.
The Magic Wallet.

The pneumonia shots are not intended to prevent most pneumonias,
Are you taking too many pills?
Don't be among the blissfully ignorant.
The concept of "Number needed to treat."
The secret of collecting nice patients.
A story about a guillotine.
Pascal's Wager
Occam's Razor

The stories and discussions are composed with references to an eclectic mix of people and works of literature including Michael Phelps, Albert Schweitzer, Ambroe Bierce, Upton Sinclair, Oscar Wilde, W.S. Gilbert, Captain Kirk, Lewis Carroll, George Takai, the Brothers Grimm, William Congreve, Dr. Lucien Leape, Dr. Norman Cousins, Calvin Coolidge, Blaise Pascal, President Ronald Reagan and and Eve the Mother of Humanity. Works referenced include Lawrence of Arabia, The Way of the World, Frankenstein, South Park, and HBO's Westworld, to name a few.

Several themes found in the book:

The studies challenging the conventional wisdom, were ignored by many doctors because they challenged conventional wisdom.

"It is difficult to get a man to understand something when his salary depends upon his not understanding it."

"You cannot have 'shared decision-making' without sharing information."

Many standard medical practices are based on promising ideas that have yet to be proven to be right.

Insulin resistance is an infrequently discussed concept which, when understood, may motivate you to lose weight even before you reach pre-diabetes.

You can't claim to be "experienced" unless you have learned something from your mistakes.

"If you knew how to put common sense into common practice, they would ask you to take over the world."

Let's Make a Deal

I need your help. I am self-publishing this book. Many highly selective *gatekeepers* in my life have let me pass through including: at Princeton University, at the University of Cincinnati College of Medicine, at my Family Medicine Residency at Akron General Medical Center (which took four of seventy applicants), the American Board of Family Practice, Hospital CEO's who hired me to be Vice President of Medical Affairs, etc. For this project, I decided to bypass the gates. I would not to put myself through the stress of finding a literary agent and a publisher. Those gatekeepers could take years and countless rejections for a first-time author who is not a celebrity. For this book I am the author, the editor, the proofreader (with help), and the marketing manager. I have tried to write clearly and I told Amazon to print the physical book in a more costly, larger than standard 7 x 10-inch format to enable a larger type font so you could more easily read it. Here's what I'm asking of you. If you think this book is of value, SPREAD THE WORD. Deal?

https://paycloseattention.net/

The Lyme Disease Detective

To give you a preview of what's coming in this book, I moved this chapter about Lyme disease to the beginning. The next chapter is the preface.

Some patients really work at better understanding their health. They actively participate in their medical care. If you are reading this book you might be one of them.

The doctor in this story had retired as the Vice President of Medical Affairs, or VPMA, at our hospital. The VPMA was the top doctor at the hospital in our 500-bed community teaching hospital. The VPMA was the doctor to whom the administration handed off all problems involving the activities of doctors. When a doctor made a mistake and a patient was harmed, the VPMA was the person who investigated. VPMA is a position I held a few years after this story took place.

As VPMA, you are super busy and have little time to see patients.

A single mistake had cost this doctor his job as the VPMA. He had gone back into practice. He had been thrown off the horse but he got right back in the saddle. You could say he was like a general who retired from leading the army and rejoined the ranks as an infantryman. I knew he had been a smart internist. I also knew he was a good man and I had hoped that going back into practice would work out well for him.

One day I saw him featured in a front-page article in the local newspaper.

The story writer wrote about a patient the doctor had helped. The reporter got involved after the family of a patient with Lyme disease had contacted her. This was no puff piece supplied to the paper by a paid publicist. Some doctors employ them, I know, but not this physician.

The patient and family were praising his good works and his skill as a physician. Lyme disease is often difficult to figure out. The article said that after seeing many other doctors who couldn't find what was wrong, the patient went to my friend, the retired VPMA, who made the diagnosis. She was now being treated and feeling better.

I saw this colleague at the hospital a few days later and I congratulated him on the nice article. He was at least 20 years my senior. He had grey hair and bushy eyebrows and when he talked to you, he looked you right in the eye. He was known to be an expert clinician. I thought I might pick up a few tips from him. I asked him, "How ever did you figure out that your patient had Lyme disease?"

He said, "It was like this: the patient said to me 'Could this be Lyme disease?' So I ran the test."

Yes, I think he was a great doctor. He was the first person to make the diagnosis because he listened to the ideas of a thinking patient and it didn't matter that it wasn't his idea to begin with. ☼

Be curious. Be skeptical! Ask questions.

To best participate in your medical care you need some learning and study, but rest assured that a lot of what's in the field of medicine is not intellectually difficult so don't be intimidated. Take your ideas to the doctor. Schedule time for this process. Schedule an extra visit if you need to.

When patients came in with an insightful idea I learned to say, "That's a good thought." And then sometimes to myself, I'd say, "My training and experience allowed me to recognize a good idea, even if I didn't think of it myself."

Table of Contents

Dedication

I would like to dedicate this work to those who promote and protect the rights of patients, especially the right to be informed, the right to meaningfully participate in decisions about their healthcare, and their right to be free from harm due to medical errors.

You know who you are.

Acknowledgements

I would like to thank the following readers who reviewed all or parts of my manuscript and made hundreds of helpful suggestions.

Mark Pugliese, J.D. Mark's sharp eye and incredible mind found many stylistic and grammatical errors, even as he groaned at my bad jokes.

Barb Steibling, R.N. I worked with Barb when she was a nurse with a state quality improvement organization in 2006-7. She "gets" what medical care should be. She read and critiqued many points in the book.

Ray Ollwerther, retired managing editor Princeton Alumni Weekly. Ray provided encouragement that my writing style was worthy of my topic.

Wm. F. Haning, III, MD, DFASAM, DLFAPA Professor Emeritus of Psychiatry Program Director, Addiction Psychiatry/Addiction Medicine John A. Burns School of Medicine, University of Hawai`i, President, American Society of Addiction Medicine. Bill provided excellent information for my chapter on addiction.

Fatimah Deffaa, Founder of the first women's bank in Saudi Arabia for Citibank Riyadh. Fatimah provided me with great encouragement and I used her knowledge to better understand Muslim culture in that chapter.

Ron Liss, American Patient Rights Association President. I sent a copy of the manuscript to Ron because I thought that in his position, he would provide perspective. I was thrilled by his support.

Adele Deeter, my "way above average" sister who does not want me to call her brilliant, helped me by spending countless hours listening to ideas as I developed them for the book.

Jan Krawczyk. Although she was a high school classmate, she and I never met until our 55th reunion. She graciously read my chapters and provided feedback. I wanted the viewpoint of a lay reader who was not biased by knowing me.

Jane Fremon, a trailblazer in Women's swimming at Princeton and an educator who founded Princeton Friend's School. She is a person who practices what she teaches and I very much appreciate her support and critique.

Chip Deffaa is an author, award-winning playwright, jazz historian, songwriter, director, and producer of plays and musical recordings. Chip's enthusiastic support was much valued.

Jim Koch, founder and brewer of Sam Adams Beer and Chairman of Boston Beer Company. Jim provided encouragement at a critical time for me.

Lenny Lepola, photographer. Using modern camera technology, Lenny took the action-stopping swimming shot on the back cover which recreated the photos described in my "Nighttime Swim at Princeton" story.

Geoff Strauss, J.D. Geoff also provided support and feedback on several chapters.

Susan Hill. Susan read several chapters and provided valuable feedback.

James Ritter, a Financial Advisor and world-record-holding masters swimmer. James made me realize my book could make a difference in people's lives and his encouragement gave me the impetus to get the book finished.

Erin Jahnke, schoolteacher. I was looking for someone younger to read the book and tell me if it would resonate. Erin, who teaches elementary school, provided that feedback.

James Purdie a superbright and super-fast masters swimmer who found 2 pages of typos in the first edition for me.

And finally, I thank my wife who prefers to remain unnamed. She continues to be the secret of my family's success.

The book has a website:

https://paycloseattention.net/

About the Author

Robert Sinsheimer, M.D. is a graduate of Princeton University where he majored in English, and achieved an All-American ranking in Swimming. He received his M.D. from the University of Cincinnati College of Medicine and chose the specialty of Family Practice. During 20 of his 42 years of practice, he held hospital medical staff leadership roles which included the responsibility for investigating the errors of a staff of hundreds of doctors. That experience provided him with a unique perspective about problems with the healthcare system. He realized that encouraging patient involvement in medical decision-making could help in a major way. Now retired, in addition to writing and swimming, he leads his local AARP tax group, providing free tax preparation to low-income seniors.

Preface

I am a retired Family Physician. Like many people who enjoy reading books, I always thought writing one would be nifty. The only problem was I didn't have anything to write about. Realizing that there were already too many books being published every year, I thought I'd be better off just doctoring. I never tried to write a book.

But in the last few years of practice, a lot of my patients said, "You should write a book." That was easy for *them* to say.

Finally, after 42 years in the profession, I retired. I missed helping people. So I started writing. I wrote about what I know, about stories from life, about funny things patients told me or said, or about thoughts that came bubbing to the surface of my mind when I was doing other things.

The result is this collection of stories and essays.

Some people like complex reading material - books that you have to read more than once before you understand the point. They don't mind a 300-page treatise on a single topic.

Here you will find fairly short stories and essays. Plus a few jokes that might make a point. I hope that if you read a chapter more than once, it is because you want to, not because you need to.

I remember when I was a kid we learned it is very difficult to put six saltines in your mouth and swallow them. They fit all right. But they swell up with saliva and form a big ball of...well you get the idea it was too big and round to go down.

I hope you will find my essays like small easy bites rather than portions that are too big. I want to fill your mind with easy-to-swallow bites.

My small essay bites will be like a single saltine. Instead of the saltine attracting the saliva, I hope that my thoughts will attract your thoughts, mix together, and then expand. It's your choice whether to swallow or not.

I would be surprised if you agree with everything I have to say.

Some chapters are very short. I have tried to make each four pages or less.

Some are stories, some jokes, and some present an ironic point of view. Some present logical conclusions about approaching your medical care. Some have an emotional content.

I may let you know my interpretation of what my stories mean, but feel free to make your own interpretation. From this book, you might learn something that will save your life or the life of someone in your family. Or not. Or, not yet.

I put a lot of things in this book that lay people often don't know, won't know, but might need to know.

Someone might say, "Why tell stories? Why not just say what you want to say."

If I did that I could list all my points on five pages. Nobody could stand to read it, though. I learned some time ago I should not just state a bunch of facts when trying to communicate concepts. The best practice is to use stories to illustrate ideas. People would miss the point when you just state what you want to say. ☼

"Just the facts ma'am" is for the detective shows.

☼

In this book, when you see this little icon that looks like the sun ☼, that's me saying you just read something that many people may not know. The symbol means I just made a point.

Pay Close Attention to That Man Behind the Curtain

It was summer, I was just about to turn 16, and my friend was 17. We were both dedicated competitive swimmers. We swam in the cool summer mornings with our AAU team at the 7 a.m. practice, we swam the noon practice at the local club pool, and we returned to our club pool after dinner to work on stroke and turns. This story happened at the end of that summer.

We were at one of the last swimming meets of the season. Our races were done for the evening. In our part of the country, summer meets are held outdoors. Almost always. This meet was at a local high school pool. It was the only meet of the summer that wasn't outdoors.

When you find yourself indoors at a summer swim meet, you are generally in the locker room, changing into or out of your suit. That is a distinction that would not appear to be terribly important to understand...yet.

All the better swimmers from two counties were there. It was the Cincinnati area-wide Junior Olympics meet. The school system was nice enough to rent out their indoor pool. In our part of the country, high school pools are all indoors.

My friend and I were hashing over the events we had swum. We were in an open area near the lockers. About 40 feet away the officials were lining up the girls for the relays at the end of the night.

A ton of swimmers had come to this meet and the lockers were overcrowded, so we had put our street clothes in our swim bags and ditched the bags in this open area, as did many other swimmers. Girls were all around. They weren't paying attention to us and my friend was not paying attention to them.

As we talked and toweled ourselves dry, he looked down at the clothes in his swim bag. He took off his bathing suit and continued to dry off, forgetting he was not in the locker room!

My friend was a brilliant young man; four years later he finished college close to the top of his Ivy League college class. He went on to medical school and became an erudite physician. Many highly intelligent people with academic skills can focus so deeply on a task or a conversation that they become unmindful of their surroundings. Such was my friend's state of mind at that moment.

No one seemed to have noticed he was naked. It took me about 10 seconds to realize what had happened. My eyes grew wide and in a somewhat loud whisper I said, "You took off your Speedo?"

He looked around. His reaction was instinctive and immediate. In a loud voice he cried out, "GIRLS DON'T LOOK!" Suddenly, of course, everyone stopped what they were doing and looked. It was a moment that went down in the local swimming lore, at least for a few days.

I am and I was an empathetic person, not that I really understood at age 15 what that word meant. I was feeling profound embarrassment for him.

But I will admit it was funny later. Like five minutes later.

When I think back to that night, it reminds me of a scene in the Wizard of Oz. Dorothy and company finally find the Wizard, who is very scary. Toto pulls on the curtain, revealing a funny-looking old man, busy operating a control panel complete with dials, switches, and levers. The old man cries into his microphone, "Pay no attention to that man behind the curtain." At that moment Dorothy, the Tin Woodsman, the Cowardly Lion, and the Scarecrow all walk over and pay very close attention.

Dorothy and the others had discovered that the magic of Oz wasn't quite so mysterious after all. Once she had seen the man behind the curtain, Dorothy quickly grasped the truth about the Wizard.

The thesis of a number of essays in this book: in your medical care you will encounter figurative curtains hiding important truths that you need to better understand.

Your Life in Five Words

Someone said everyone should try to describe what they do in life in five words. My five words as a Family Doctor: "Help patients make smarter decisions."

If you are missing critical information, how can you make the smartest decision?

I have learned that confidential negotiations involve three levels. First, we have the people in the conference room. They know what is being discussed and what is at stake. Second, we have the people *just outside* the room. They know that decisions are being made inside that will affect them. They want to be "in the know" but they are not allowed in the room. Third, we have the people walking by in the hallway or out on the street. What happens behind those closed doors affects them too, but they don't even know there is a meeting going on.

When you are in that second level, you know there is some important information behind the door. You are on the wrong side of the door, hoping to hear something - looking at the curtain before Toto pulls it open in the Wizard of Oz analogy. Later on you can privately ask one of the in-the-room people what went on. And they might tell you.

But if you are the blissfully ignorant passerby in the third level, you don't have a clue what's going on in the negotiation room because you don't even know there is a negotiation.

If you don't see the curtain, how can you ask what's behind it?

"Help patients make smarter decisions" is a tall order.

Never Expect Someone to Make a Change In Their Life Unless You Give Them an Adequate Reason to Do So.

As a doctor, I gained a certain perspective. Every doctor has this experience: "What a sad thing for that patient! If he/she had only done X earlier then Y would not have happened."

"You need to take MUCH better control of your diabetes," I said to a patient when I was a young doctor. The patient said "No thank you, I feel fine," and found a new doctor. Three years later I read her name in the newspaper. In the obituary section. Neglected diabetes is very risky.

I thought it was my job to try to persuade patients to do what was in their best interests. It sounds simple and kind of obvious.

As I just mentioned in the prior essay, someone wrote that everyone should try to describe their job in five or six words. I came up with "Help patients make smarter decisions."

To each patient, I gave the best advice I could give. But a lot of the time, even though I knew patients needed to change something in their lives, they did not change.

I didn't "get it." I had spent 11 years of my life in college, medical school, and residency just so I could give my patients this great advice, and then I'd sadly watch what went wrong when they didn't follow it.

I was unhappy and frustrated in these situations.

As the years of practice passed, I was fascinated by this question: Why don't patients make lifestyle changes that would be in their best interest? Lose weight! Exercise! Drink less! Don't smoke! I knew it wasn't easy, but look at what's at stake.

Oscar Wilde said something like this (I modernized it a bit): "To keep from getting old, I'd do anything except stop smoking, quit drinking, lose weight, and exercise."

I remember this dialogue in the play "The Way of the World," written in 1700 by William Congreve. The character Mirabel reveals to his friend Fainall that he is aware of his lover's flaws but those defects haven't altered his attraction to her. In fact, he says he has become used to her faults, made an extensive list of them, learned to tolerate them, and in fact feels that, in time, he will like her faults as much as he likes his own:

> And for a discerning man somewhat too passionate a lover, for I like her with all her faults; nay, like her for her faults. Her follies are so natural, or so artful, that they become her, and those affectations which in another woman would be odious serve but to make her more agreeable. I'll tell thee, Fainall, she once used me with that insolence that in revenge I took her to pieces, sifted her, and separated her failings: I studied 'em and got 'em by rote. The catalog was so large that I was not without hopes, one day or other, to hate her heartily. To which end I so used myself to think of 'em, that at length, contrary to my design and expectation, they gave me every hour less and less disturbance, till in a few days it became habitual to me to remember 'em without being displeased. They are now grown as familiar to me as my own frailties, and in all probability in a little time longer I shall like 'em as well.

11

Of course! I get it! It's funny! That's it. They won't change because people enjoy their bad habits! The nice thing about studying literature is that good fiction is about human nature.

I wonder why we call them "bad" habits if we like them so much!

That's why patients did not give up eating too much, being inactive, smoking, etc.! If I wanted healthier patients, which I really did, I needed to sell them on reasons to give up the bad habits they enjoyed in exchange for better ones they could also enjoy. ☼

Sometimes I wanted to scream: "If you could see what I have seen, you would change!!!!!" But screaming bothers all the other patients in the office. I only did that in the office once. That's in a later chapter.

I couldn't scream it. I needed to sell it. I needed to provide the patient with good enough reasons to change.

Did that work? Sometimes it did. More often it did not.

So I had to develop a philosophy for patients who would not follow good advice: it doesn't matter how many fish swim away, it only matters how many you catch. At the same time, I worked on my sales pitch.

How to sell ideas? One way is a story. I learned when possible it is better to tell the message in a story than to spew out instructions and facts. I kept trying to make my stories better. That's where some of the chapters in this book originated.

NEVER EXPECT SOMEONE TO MAKE A CHANGE IN THEIR LIFE UNLESS YOU GIVE THEM AN ADEQUATE REASON TO DO SO. And that means presenting that reason in a way they can understand and remember.

The Magic Wallet

"Try to convince patients to replace bad habits they enjoy with better habits they can also enjoy." With that in mind, I invented the Magic Wallet.

The best part of exercise is feeling very relaxed for the rest of the day and having more energy the next day.

I took a 22 year break between college swimming and Masters swimming. My excuse was medical school, residency, starting a practice, and kids. In those inactive years, I thought exercise was walking out to the mailbox or taking the stairs instead of the elevator. I distinctly remember something that happened a few weeks before I started swimming again.

My 9-year-old son had joined the YMCA swim team that year and I was picking him up after practice that evening. He got into the car and plopped into the seat. He said, "I feel dead!" Then he paused. He added, "I feel great!"

Something clicked. I bought a swimsuit and a pair of goggles and joined the Y. Swimming became my main exercise. Three decades later, I'm still swimming four or five times a week.

I would tell my patients about the Magic Wallet, a concept I made up to illustrate a point about exercise.

The Magic Wallet is an ordinary-looking wallet containing $100. As the day goes on you spend money on this or that and when you put the wallet on the bureau and go to sleep there is only $85 left. But when you wake up, you find $100 magically back in the wallet again. Every day the wallet replenishes itself as you sleep.

Magic wallets are really wonderful, aren't they?

Now here is an even better feature. If you spend $80 out of your $100 in one day, really depleting the magic wallet, you will only have $20 left when you fall to sleep. But when you wake up there's now $101 in the magic wallet. Not $100. Yes, a dollar extra! You see, every day you drain the wallet, there's going to be even more money the next morning. It gradually builds up. Pretty soon you have $200.

Patients would say, "I'd love one of those!"

I'd say, "You have one."

You see, there is no such thing as a magic wallet for money. But your muscles and your energy supply act like a magic wallet. The more you drain them each day, the more energy you have the next day. Everyone has a magic energy wallet and most people don't think of it.

When patients told me they were too tired to exercise, I told them, "Maybe you are tired because you don't exercise." ☼ Then I told them about the Magic Wallet. I'd advise to start off slow.

Feeling relaxed and having more energy are the most satisfying parts of exercise. Health benefits are just byproducts.

How To Make Patients More Curious To Learn What They Should Know But Don't?

Answer: give them permission to ask questions and encourage them to be curious. Not enough patients have the burning desire to learn the facts which help in choosing from the options the doctor advises.☼ This is an important paragraph. Read it again.

How do we make patients more curious so they can learn enough to "get it," to incorporate into their belief systems

14

those "adequate reasons to change?" Often it's not just a simple "if A, then B" situation. Can we discover factors C, D, E, etc. that also affect the decision-making?

Maybe we need to help identify the barriers that stop people from doing better. Maybe it's an elaborate hairstyle that stops the woman from exercising. She can't squeeze in a 30 minute workout if it takes 20 minutes to dry her hair. Maybe it's a cramped kitchen that stops the patient from preparing better foods. Maybe they know they cannot afford fresh vegetables or fruit but they never learned that frozen vegetables and fruit are equal nutritionally.☼ Thank you Clarence Birdseye (1886-1956) for being the pioneer of frozen foods. You changed the world.

As in many fields, only when we peel back the layers of the onion can we help the patient understand which decision is best for them.

When patients get smarter they ask more questions. Good doctors will listen. They may realize from the questions patients ask that what they were about to tell the patient does not fit that patient. The patient's questions prompt a better understanding of the patient.

As I wrote in a previous chapter when patients came in with an insightful idea I learned to say, "That's a good thought." And then sometimes to myself, I'd say, "My training and experience allow me to recognize a good idea, even if I didn't think of it myself." Like the Lyme disease detective.

By the way, "Because I said so - I'm a doctor," is not an adequate reason for making changes.

Next, I'll discuss a single example of giving an adequate reason.

"Pneumonia Shots Is a Bad Name For It"

Here is a simple "secret" most people have not learned. It's simple if you can define the words. If you don't know the difference in the words, it's confusing to people. Here's the "secret:" We don't give the "Pneumonia Shot" to prevent pneumonia.

That' not the main reason.

Let's define terms. Actually, it is not a "pneumonia shot." It is properly called the "Pneumococcal Vaccine" because it is designed to help the body resist one really dangerous germ known as S. Pneumoniae or pneumococcus.

A famous doctor, Sir William Osler, called pneumococcus "The Captain of the Men of Death." This bacterium causes a lot of different infections, and pneumonia is just one of them. The pneumococcus can spread through the body rapidly and create a condition known as sepsis.

"Sepsis" is another term needing to be defined. That's an infection that starts to overcome the entire body and its critical systems: lungs, liver, kidneys, brain, and heart and is fatal in a day or two if not treated soon enough. Not uncommonly, advanced sepsis kills the patient even after treatment with the right antibiotic. And plain old penicillin kills pneumococcus very nicely.

The reason we advise pneumococcal immunization is to prevent pneumococcal sepsis. ☼ I think we say to patients it to prevent "pneumonia" because it's simpler to explain.

That simplification causes confusion because Pneumococcal Vaccine does not immunize against most cases of pneumonia. Why? The kind of pneumonia that most people would get is caused by viruses and bacteria other than pneumococcus. The pneumococcal vaccine does not help our immune system fight the other bacterial species or viruses.

Patients would tell me, "I got the Pneumonia Shot and then I got pneumonia anyway." They think the immunization did not work. We hear, "Well my friend had that vaccine twice and still came down with pneumonia."

Other people resist the immunization, thinking, "I don't worry about pneumonia. I've known a lot of people who had pneumonia and they did alright." Yes, people with non-pneumococcal pneumonia without sepsis generally recover.

Other patients will develop these other types of pneumonia and get sick enough to need treatment. But some of them stay away. In their minds, they ignore the evidence that they could have pneumonia. "I didn't dream I could have had pneumonia, Doctor. Don't you know, I had the shot for that?

For years this vaccine was very underutilized. A 2014 CDC study for people over age 64 with no underlying conditions found only 42% of eligible adult patients had received this vaccine. For people with four or more chronic, high-risk conditions, only 79% of patients had received it.

How common is pneumococcal sepsis? If you hate numbers, you can skip to the two sentences in bold. With a big push to improve immunization rates, the attack rate for this type of sepsis has fallen from 59 cases per year per 100,000 in 1998 to 23 per 100,000 in the year 2015. Let's calculate: 100,000 divided by 59 is about 1700. Before the push to improve vaccination rates, one in 1700 Americans was getting this type of sepsis each year. Using a little mental math, we saved 59 cases minus 23 cases = 36 cases per 100,000 per year which is about 1 in 2800. But only about half of the population took the vaccine so we might have saved 72 not 36 if everybody got the immunization. 100k divided by 72 is 1,400. **So giving 1,400 immunizations could save one life from sepsis every year**.

It's more complicated than this because giving the vaccine to all children has also helped reduce the attack rate in the over 64 age group. The kids are less likely to spread it to the older members of the family. But if we consider over a span of 10 years, giving 1,400 immunization would save 10 cases of sepsis. **That's one case prevented in 140 people immunized over 10 years.** That makes immunization against the pneumococcal bacterium even more appealing.

For those readers who have a policy of skipping over anything with math in it, here's the short version. Assuming everyone gets a sore arm from the pneumococcal vaccine, and that's an exaggeration, which would you rather do to your patients? Produce 140 sore arms from giving the vaccine or skip the shots and miss the chance to save one patient in those 140 from dying prematurely?

So, armed with those numbers, I can tell the hesitant patient one of my stories: "Some years ago I saw a nice lady not much different from you, who spent a month in intensive care on a ventilator with pneumococcal sepsis, the very condition this shot blocks. She was treated by all the smartest specialists with a ton of the right medications and then she died anyway from that pneumococcal infection. Before she got sepsis she looked normal and healthy. Her death was miserable and prolonged. Let me tell you: I'd rather give 140 shots than watch one lady die. Let's give you the vaccine today."

In the next essay, I describe a similar situation that is more complex and also more important.

Why Have So Few Patients Been Told About Insulin Resistance?

A patient goes to the doctor. The doctor says, "You're too fat." The patient says: "I'd like a second opinion." The doctor says, "Your hair is cut too short."

My message to doctors: "You're too fat" is not how to bring up this topic.

My message to patients: the doctor's not talking about how you look, it's about insulin resistance.

It's a reality that affects two-thirds of the U.S. population and leads to the #1 cause of death, heart disease, and the #5 cause of death, stroke. This is the problem of insulin resistance. It might be your adequate reason for making a change if you only knew what it was.

In a sentence: Fat accumulating around the middle increases the body's production of insulin, which leads to more heart attacks and strokes, even before diabetes is reached.

Pull back the curtain. We see "Insulin Resistance."

Have you never heard this? It's not exactly easy to find by googling. It's a bit complicated to explain. So I'll try to make it as easy as ABCDE.

Terms and concepts:

Insulin is a hormone made by the pancreas that helps the body regulate (lower) blood sugar. It helps sugar get into the cells where it is needed. It also makes you hungry.

Fat around the middle (your waist) somehow interferes with how insulin works. You need more to get the job done. That's called **resistance**.

The body compensates for the weaker insulin effect by increasing the production of insulin. Like with money, as prices rise, if the money buys less with inflation you need more money to stay even. Extra insulin production allows

19

the body to keep the blood glucose nearly normal so you get an acceptable fasting blood glucose at your physical. Or you might just see a very slightly elevated fasting blood glucose on your yearly physical. All is good, right? Good work, see you next year.

Wrong! Elevated insulin levels promote atherosclerosis, the process by which plaque forms inside your arteries. Atherosclerosis leads to stroke and heart attack. When your cells start resisting insulin, the pancreas copes by making more insulin. That delays the diagnosis of diabetes because the much higher insulin levels mostly compensate for the resistance. It becomes a vicious cycle: as the weight increases, the insulin loses effectiveness and the body makes more but the insulin makes you hungry so you have more trouble losing weight. Goodness gracious! (That's how a polite person curses.)

Yeah, remember that higher insulin levels make you hungry. That's why restaurants served rolls before you ordered. The bread provokes insulin secretion and you get hungry when you are ordering. Better for the restaurant.

During these years of higher insulin production, the arteries are developing plaque or "hardening." And this starts years before you get diagnosed with type 2 diabetes.

Review ABCDE: increasing fat on your waist (A) causes insulin resistance (B) which causes excess production of insulin (C) which increases appetite. Elevated insulin causes atherosclerosis (D) which causes increased rates of heart attack and stroke (E).

For people really into brevity: A->B->C->D->E or even shorter: Fat around the middle causes heart attack and stroke.

You don't need to measure insulin levels. You just measure your waist around the umbilicus. It should be under 40 for men and under 35 for women. Or have the doctor check a fasting blood glucose. If you are overweight and your FBG is nearly 100 or over, you very likely have insulin resistance.

Insulin resistance plays a significant role in the pathogenesis of other serious medical conditions as well, including obesity, hypertension, type 2 diabetes, dyslipidemia, and cardiovascular disease. The growing obesity epidemic in the United States continues to escalate the number of individuals at risk for developing insulin resistance, From: https://www.pharmacytimes.com/publications/issue/2012/october2012/insulin-resistance-recognizing-the-hidden-danger Olatunbosun ST. Insulin resistance. Medscape website. http://emedicine.medscape.com/article/122501-overview.

Diabetes mellitus. Merck Manual for Healthcare Professionals Online Edition. www.merckmanuals.com/professional/endocrine_and_metabolic_disorders/diabetes_mellitus_and_disorders_of_carbohydrate_metabolism/diabetes_mellitus_dm.html.]

In medical school, I had a mentor who told me, "Never tell a patient to lose weight. They never lose anyway, and if you tell them that they will hate you for mentioning it and you will hate them for not losing."

This was a doctor?

So let's say a doctor tells the patient, "You need to lose ten pounds." Let me tell you, that rarely works. This is now the 1000th time they were told to lose weight and 996 of those times it was the patient talking to himself.

The patients get offended because they think you are attacking how they look. Overweight people don't look bad to me. They look like everybody else. It's not about looks.

Let's expose "insulin resistance" for what it is. It's the most important reason why getting fat around the middle could rob you of your health.

I should not fail to mention the effect an extra 30 pounds may have on your knees and hips.

21

With less risk of being misunderstood, you can tell the patient, "You have insulin resistance, which increases your chance of getting a heart attack or a stroke. Type 2 diabetes is the next step for you if you don't lose some fat around the middle."

No, that's just stating the facts. In one ear and out the other. Maybe use a "handout" with this essay or something similar.

How Did I Lose 30 Pounds?

When I stepped on the scale one day it said 203 pounds. I had weighed 166 pounds in college and that was when I was much more muscular. I did not like 203. I resolved to get serious. Within a year I lost 30 pounds. I've gained three back but I'm OK.

My fasting blood sugar had been just short of prediabetes and now I'm normal. My kidney function had been borderline and that's normal now. My knees were aching a lot. No longer do I sleep with the pillow between my knees. How did I lose the weight?

First I must state that everybody needs to find what works for them. This is what worked for me.

See my later chapter on Optimism.

But here are some ideas that helped me. If I start to put on pounds I follow these rules again.

At some point, you need to keep a diary and record everything you eat. I did that for the first three months. It's a real bother but it's essential. I measured the number of grams of everything I ate and calculated the calories of each item. I recorded each thing I ate on a Libre Office spreadsheet. As a result, I developed a rough idea of how many calories are in what I eat as long as I weigh the portion.

Use a reliable food scale and weigh your portions even if you are not calculating your calories. It helps to get to know the size of your portions to avoid portion creep.

Recording what I ate and figuring out the total number of calories per day helped me stay on track. I did not set a rigid limit on calories per day. I just watched each day as the daily calorie count climbed and let my sense of responsibility to my body take it from there.

From the Pirates of Penzance, lyrics by W.S. Gilbert:

Fredrick: "You don't mean to say you are going to hold me to that?"

King: "No, we merely remind you of the fact, and leave the rest to your sense of duty."

Eat about the same number of calories every day. It's much easier to eat that way. Having a "cheat day" is popular with people trying to lose weight, but it makes things harder for two or three days after that.

If I have been hungry too long, I always eat a little something between meals. You will discover the best snacks with the fewest calories that will suppress the hunger for the longest time until the next meal.

Cereal with milk makes a great snack, but always weigh the cereal. It can turn out to be very high in calories when you just eyeball the amount.

Sauces add flavor to bland, healthy foods. If you have time you can make sauces but it's quicker to buy them. How do you weigh the amount of sauce you add to a dish? You put the jar on the food scale and tare it to zero. After you add the sauce to your food weigh the jar again. How much you used shows as a negative number. You need a scale that doesn't power off for at least a minute to do this. I had one that would power off after 15 seconds of inactivity and that was no good. I'd put the container back on the scale and it had shut off.

Don't eat unless you are hungry, or another way of saying it: resolve to never eat just for pleasure.

If you really like to eat for pleasure, and that's about everybody, remember that when you start to lose weight everything tastes great. So just have a bite of that cake and freeze the rest. I bought a Costco chocolate cake recently and soon had 12 pieces of cake frozen in quart zip-lock bags. I might defrost one a week. I'm thinking about cake tonight.

Then I remember since I'm cutting down calories, maybe half an apple, which tastes so extra good now, will do the trick. I mean they're both great, right? Remember to focus on those great tastes of plain food.

After you eat, give it time to work. It might take half an hour for that hunger to subside.

An hour of hunger isn't the worst thing in the world, and it's harder to notice it when you are busy.

I like to consume two cups of coffee per day. I use decaf. I buy green coffee beans and roast them at home in my garage. That's another story. But coffee helps reduce the risk of several types of cancer.

If you need to sweeten your coffee, it's possible you are trying to drink bitter coffee. It could get that way if you brew it over 203 degrees F. If you brew coffee under 193 it will be under-extracted so you start to use more and that can make it bitter. Don't use too much coffee. Use the scale for measuring that and check the temp of the water coming out of your drip coffeemaker.

Keep a glass of good-tasting water out all day.

Don't use artificial sweeteners or diet soda pop. They just condition your mind to expect sweet things all the time.

Eat enough high-protein foods. I do eat meat but I favor the leaner types. Top round is much leaner than ribeye. White chicken, not dark. Before I cook ground beef I slice it umpteen times on a cutting board to make it more spoonable after cooking and then I brown it in the instant pot on the sauté setting. Deep in the instant pot, it does not splatter grease. Then I pour it through the plastic strainer to lose as much fat as I can.

I try to eat six ounces of mixed vegetables per day, not the starchy ones like carrots, peas, lima beans, or potatoes. Think of those as the same thing as bread. That's how dietitians classify them. For my veggies, I use the kind of veggies they sell for stir fry like onion, celery, mushroom, string beans, green or red peppers etc. If it's a seed like corn or beans, it's high in starch for the growth of the new plant.

Here's a little nutritional secret: anything that grows under the ground is much higher in calories.☼ Like beets and potatoes. They make granulated sugar from beets. Carrots don't taste sugary but cook them and then taste how sweet they are. If it's underground the plant is using it to store starch.

If my wife makes some dish, I take a medium portion and then add those six ounces of vegetables. She says it's weird to do that. I have lasagna veggie casserole, beef macaroni veggie casserole, and mac and cheese veggie casserole. The veggies added only 80 calories and now I have a much nicer-sized portion.

To make a low-calorie dinner entrée, think how an Asian restaurant makes meals. They have four ingredients - the protein, the veggies, the rice, and the sauce. With four different proteins like shrimp, chicken, beef, and tofu and four different sauces such as Sweet and Sour, General Tso, Teriyaki, and Peanut you now have 16 different meals you can concoct. If you watch the size of the rice and meat portions and the amount of sauce, the calories in such a meal are fewer than you would think.

Use fruit for a snack but don't overload on that. By the way, a few drops of lemon juice on half an apple will keep it looking good overnight.

Don't worry about the fats in healthy foods like avocado and nuts. I mean eat them, but still measure how much. I consume seven grams of pistachios every day. I enjoy one at a time with my coffee. The nuts are better for me than a sweet pastry.

I can be happy without alcohol. But if you drink don't forget to count that too. It can add up.

Use the lower calorie sauces or salad dressings; there are plenty that have only 30 to 45 calories in two tablespoons. Put the salad dressing bottle on the digital scale and tare it. Pour a little on the salad. Re-weigh the bottle. The scale shows you how much you used as a negative number. Using an oversize bowl to mix the salad and the dressing can help make a little dressing go further. Don't confuse low fat with low calories. When you check the label you often find that the "Low Fat" product has the same or more calories per portion, due to containing more carbs. Carbohydrates break down faster and that stimulates insulin which makes you hungrier.

Calculate the calories in some of your favorite meals and more often choose entrees you like as much but which have fewer calories.

Remember, you may lose seven pounds in the first ten days but in those first ten days that's just less poop inside your colon. A pound of fat from your middle is worth 3,500 calories. Losing a pound a week over the long haul is very good. That's a deficit of 500 calories per day. That's a lot. But that's 25 pounds in a half a year.

If you are inactive due to arthritis, for example, and simply can't do more, it will take a longer time to lose weight. It will be hard to have a deficit of 250 calories in a day if your body only needs 1,200 to keep your weight steady.

Finally, you might need to put some foods on the "Do Not Touch" list. For me, it's peanut butter, chips, soda pop, and sour cream.

I knew a very old doctor who told me, "Here's a simple diet. If you like it don't eat it, but if you don't like it, eat as much as you like." (That won't work, it's a joke.)

A good goal for you? Check with your doctor but one idea is to try to get your BMI into the normal range. Just below overweight. It may not be good to be thin as a rail when you get to be 65.

Very muscular people will have a higher BMI despite being lean, so take that in to consideration. ☼

The Grandmother and Her Grandson

Early one morning, a grandmother was walking along the beach with her four-year-old grandson. The boy was decked out in a nice jacket with matching shorts and a little white hat. They were looking for shells. No one noticed the huge wave forming out on the ocean, the one that was ten feet tall, very dark, and bearing down on them.

The wave crashed over the two and when the waters receded the grandmother looked around and could not find her grandson. She looked out over the ocean and up and down the beach, but there was no sign of him.

She desperately raised her hands up to the heavens and cried out, "Lord, please bring back my grandson! He's just an innocent child. If you must have someone, take me, I'm just a useless old woman."

Soon another wave formed out on the water. This wave was larger and even darker and it rolled in towards the shore where the grandmother stood waiting to accept God's will. The wave crashed over her and she was completely enveloped by the ocean.

When the waters receded, she was still standing and a few feet away stood her little grandson.

She ran over to check him and found he was fine, no broken bones, no bruises. He wasn't even choking on the seawater. He was just very wet. She held her arms up to the heavens and she cried out, "Lord? He was wearing a hat!!!!"

Choose To Be Grateful Or Be a Complainer

Part of feeling good and healthy is a positive attitude and a sense of being thankful. A few years ago I learned the definition of a word that had escaped me up to that point in life: kvetch. It's a Yiddish word that has become popular in recent decades. A kvetch is a person who complains a great deal.

Why would some people complain endlessly? I heard an explanation based on folklore. American Yiddish immigrants believed that the Devil looks for people to ruin and is most highly interested in ruining happy people. He doesn't look so hard for people who are already unhappy or disadvantaged. So if you simply complain all day, the Devil will not realize how good you have it and will go elsewhere.

This idea ties into the breaking of the glass at the Jewish wedding. That is supposed to symbolize the destruction of the Temple in Jerusalem. The glass is wrapped up in a napkin and the groom's foot does the honors. But according to this "let's not attract the Devil" idea, a wedding where an expensive crystal wine glass is broken is no longer a perfect one. That will keep the evil one looking somewhere else.

I don't subscribe to this philosophy. I think being thankful in life is healthier than constantly finding something to complain about. If I were in pain six hours out of every day that would be bad, yes. But if I feel much better the other 18 hours, I should try to be thankful for that.

Your body is a gift from God. If you think of it that way, you will take better care of it. If you think your body is a piece of junk, you might figure: "Why bother?"

This negativity can lead to what people call "self-fulfilling prophesies."

Think of your body as junk and it may turn into junk due to your neglect.

I often need to remind myself of another problem that comes from negativity: perfectionism. Something inside tells you, "Everything has to be right. Anything else is wrong."

Why do we focus on the little defects in things and people? About 20 years ago I learned the mantra, "Don't let the perfect get in the way of the good." If you wait for perfect things or perfect people in life, you will be waiting a long time.

I had a fortune cookie that made me laugh: "You will never be a top dog if you growl all the time."

Are You Taking Too Many Pills?

You might be. Many doctors spend more time on what new medication you might need and less thought about what med you can safely stop taking. When you lose weight and keep it off is a good time to ask the doctor whether you can stop something. You might not need as many meds for hypertension. You might not need that NSIAD arthritis pill for your knees. NSAIDs are hard on the kidneys and the stomach as we get older so they are good ones to think about dropping. It's important to bring this up unless you and your doctor have already been working on reducing your medications.

You might ask your doctor to run your meds through a drug interaction program to see if there are any serious conflicts. I'd recommend doing that yourself at home but....there are so many interactions that are trivial but will be listed...the results are usually overwhelming. It's difficult for the layman to separate the important from the unimportant interactions. So if you find a drug interaction program online, just don't get bent out of shape by the minor interactions, but bring the printout to your doctor if you have a printer.

What's your doctor thinking when you ask what med you could stop? Sometimes she/he's thinking, "If I stop drug X and the patient gets worse it will be a mess. I'd better not rock the boat."

That's why you need to keep asking.

I used to kid around with the medical students, "Just remember, you get paid the same for stopping a medication as you do for starting one."

It is definitely work for the doctor to do this. After dropping something, he/she may want you to come back in a month to see if you are really stable without that medication you had taken for years.

Don't stop meds on your own though. It's risky to do that. I can certainly recall patients who rebelled by stopping everything and a few of them actually looked fine. But even though someone looks fine a week after stopping medication, things might go bad two weeks after that.

But I Don't Need to Know That Stuff

Since people do the opposite, maybe instead of "GIRLS DON"T LOOK!" we should yell "PATIENT'S DON'T LOOK!" Or maybe, "PAY NO ATTENTION TO THE FACTS!"

I want to shed light on some of the underappreciated facts that affect medical care choices. I also want to provide insights that might help patients understand better reasons to take good care of themselves.

I think that to be healthy in a profit-driven healthcare system, the patient needs to develop a persistent curiosity blended with a dose of polite skepticism. "Show me the 'Why?' don't just tell me what to do."

The patient who lacks the facts is at a disadvantage. You thought that pretty curtain along the wall was for decoration but maybe there's a little man behind it who is manipulating what you see. In many critical medical decisions, you don't get the right answers if you don't even know which questions to ask.

You might think: "I don't need to know that stuff now. I'll figure it out when I need to, right?"

In medical school, I learned to say "Hmmm." I would reply: "Hmmm, I'm not so sure about that. You want to find out why losing weight is uber important for your future but you tell me you will be ready to be convinced to lose weight when you need to? Like after you have the heart attack or the stroke? Like when your arthritis is so bad you have trouble exercising? That's when you are going to do the research?"

When you are well you don't work to gain an understanding of things that are in your future. For many of us, we are under-concerned with our future but we are over-concerned with garbage from the past.

A lot of patients think "I don't know that medical stuff... I'm not a doctor. I trust my doctor, he/she knows what's best for me." But doctors these days don't have the time to think of your future. To help them do that, they might need a little nudge in the form of your questions.

One type of wisdom or understanding comes through pattern recognition. Over time you have seen things. You say to yourself, "I have some experience with this situation. Been there, seen that." If you know more, you might recognize a hidden threat that is in the semi-distant future. Without that insight from experience, you don't make any changes. Ask your doctor to open up that part of his/her brain for you.

What if a specialist advised something and then you ask for all the options? The specialist tells you. How do you choose?

Maybe that's a good time to see your Family Doctor and have her/him help you sort through the facts to help you choose the best option for you.

When I recall what happened to some of my patients, I can think of many instances in which the patient would have done better if they had known or understood more about what was going on. I certainly had patients whose outcomes were changed for the better because they insisted on understanding more. Do you recall the story of the Lyme disease detective the chapter at the front of the book?

Sometimes when patients asked better questions, that made me think harder. Sometimes their tough questions made me look up and learn something I would not have known otherwise. Go for it!

The Adventure of the Unmarried Swimmer
On a Tropical Cruise

An unmarried man on a tropical cruise is taking a walk on the promenade deck early one morning. He looks out to see an island on the horizon about three miles away.

Suddenly there is a loud noise and the ship starts sinking rapidly. In 20 seconds the cruise ship is completely underwater. There is no time to launch the lifeboats.

He treads water. He looks around and sees no survivors. So he heads towards the island.

Luckily he is a strong swimmer. In under two hours, he makes it to the island.

He gets up on a rock and scans the sea. He sees another swimmer about a half-mile out.

He swims out. It's a woman and she's exhausted from the effort. He pulls her towards the island and helps her ashore. She's cold, pale, and nearly lifeless, but as he revives her, he recognizes her. She's a well-known movie star, only a few years younger than he is. She is the kind of actress who plays leading ladies in romantic roles.

You never know who's on a cruise with you!

No more survivors appear. The next day she's recovered enough to talk and they introduce themselves. They gather food and make a shelter and look out for rescue planes or ships, but none come.

Days turn into weeks. Acquaintance turns to friendship and then to romance. Luckily the island has fruits, the sea has fish and the weather is warm.

One day the two survivors, now lovers, are sitting around the campfire after dinner. He says to her: "Honey, can I ask a favor?"

"What can I do for you?" she replies.

"Would it be OK if I take a bit of cold charcoal from the fire and draw a mustache on your upper lip?"

(Reader, trust me on this story.)

"Sounds kinky, but if that's what you want, go ahead."

He gives her a mustache. He stares at her.

He says, "Could I draw a full beard?"

"Sure, whatever amuses you, we've got plenty of time."

He gives her a beard with the charcoal.

He says, "One more thing, could I call you George?"

"I guess that would be alright. OK, I'll be George."

He sits down next to her, turns to her, and says, "George!!! You'll never believe who I've been sleeping with!!!"

Byproducts of Wasting Time

I sat and listened to the patient. It was our second visit. He said, "I know what's wrong with me. I have bronchitis again. The same thing happened to me last year. Whenever I breathe in the cold air outdoors, I cough. And you know what else? The cold air makes it feel kinda tight."

This man usually went to the older doctor I had joined in practice. My partner was a good doctor; he's gone now. That day and for a prior visit, they could not fit this patient into his schedule. As the new doctor, he was mine for this visit and the time before when I saw him for something else.

On that earlier visit, I had told him a dumb joke. Something like:

The Aleutian Islands are a chain of mostly volcanic Alaskan islands extending from the mainland towards Asia.

35

Less than 10,000 people live there. I once heard about an eye doctor who moved to the Aleutian Islands. No one understood why he would move to such a remote area. It was because he wanted to become an optical Aleutian.

OR*: Do you know Forrest Gump's password?   It was 1forrest1.*

Someone taught me to tell a joke to relax the patient and try to get them to feel you weren't super rushed.

I looked at the chart. About a year ago he was in to see my partner. The record of that visit read something like: "Bronchitis, cough in cold air. Lungs clear. Heart normal. RX: Doxycycline 100 mg daily x 7 days (an antibiotic).

What did the patient tell me that was different?   He elaborated a bit more about his symptoms. He gave me the clue about how the cold air made his chest feel tight.

I told him his symptom sounded like angina, not bronchitis. I arranged for a treadmill test. He flunked it. It was strongly positive. Next, he had a heart cath. In that test the specially trained cardiologist puts a long tube or catheter into your arm or groin artery and threads it up to your heart and takes pictures of the heart's arteries. The left main coronary artery was severely blocked. If a clot were to form on that plaque, which would not be uncommon, he would probably die. He needed a bypass. He got one. He survived for over a decade.

There is no compelling medical reason to tell a joke or a story. It's only a way of saying, "If I have time to kid around for a minute, it means I like you as a person. I ALSO have time to hear that concern or symptom that you thought was not worth troubling me about (such as that funny chest tightness that only comes on in the cold air.)

Trust Your Doctor? Depends On How You Define the Words

Considering the state of the progress of modern medicine, we are very lucky to be alive at this time in history. The advances have been amazing. But not every so-called advance is great or even good. Should you place full trust in all that modern medicine offers?

Hardly. One of my colleagues said something about insurance companies which I can rephrase like this: "I trust modern medicine as far as I can drop-kick it."

My target for this book is people who admire our medical system but don't trust it and want to be smarter patients. You see, some parts of modern medical care are great and others are not so great or even hazardous for your health. How do we tell which are which? Who's our tugboat captain, keeping us from running over the hidden rocks in the harbor just below the surface?

I thought that Family Doctors would do that. I tried to do that. But I couldn't be everywhere at once. You need an involved Family Doctor but every patient needs to be his own tugboat captain too.

We start by realizing that medical truths are not black or white.

Let's look at the FDA. The FDA won't approve a drug until it has been proven safe and effective; that's their legal mandate as defined by congress. But if that new drug helps one patient in 100, that might be enough to be called effective. What you think is a useful definition of "effective" is not the same as how researchers or the FDA use the word.

Imagine if Consumer Reports said a car was reliable if it lasted 10 years *for one customer in 100.*

In other words, in the FDA universe, slightly effective or sometimes effective counts as effective. ☼

37

What about cost-effectiveness? Not in their job description. That's not their business.

"U.S. regulators, on the other hand, aren't too concerned about costs. The Food and Drug Administration considers the safety and efficacy of a drug before granting its final approval, but it doesn't look at the financial impact."

https://fortune.com/2015/02/04/is-it-time-for-the-fda-to-consider-cost-when-it-comes-to-new-drugs/

About 20 years ago my late mother, who was 82 at the time, sent me a magazine advertisement for a new treatment for sore muscles: lasers. The ad said this new laser device was FDA approved.

I was very busy as usual, but you do anything for your mother, right? I researched this treatment of sore muscles laser devices.

It was actually FDA-approved. I thought to myself: "Well I'll be damned!" I looked further.

I found the actual FDA application for the product. After poring through maybe ten pages of fine print I learned the following: The laser treatments heat up the sore muscles, ever so slightly. The effect is comparable to applying a heating pad. Apparently, FDA has found heating pads to be effective for sore muscles so they were compelled to approve the muscle-warming lasers as they were also effective.

I knew without researching further that the laser treatments would cost a lot more than your home heating pad.

Was the laser effective? Yes. I'm not impressed by heating pads but I know some people find relief with them. I worry more about the very old or very young falling asleep on them and getting a burn.

Bottom line: slightly effective = effective if you are the FDA. Cost-effective = "we don't regulate that" if you are the FDA.

By the way, you may have heard that you should not use a heating pad if you suspect appendicitis. Why is that?

Because the heating pad may relieve pain enough that you will delay medical treatment and the appendix may rupture. ☼

In summary, to an extent, you do have to trust your doctor, but you also may have to ask probing questions when he/she makes a recommendation. Think more and ask further questions. Make an extra visit if necessary if there isn't enough time.

My Patient Accidentally Swallowed Bleach

Whenever you suspect you or a member of the family took something that might be unsafe, calling poison control is the first thing to do. They have great resources.

Most people who drink bleach just take just a swig of it by accident and discover it was not what they thought they were drinking. So it's not much swallowed.

Poison Control will probably advise drinking four to eight ounces of water or milk to dilute it. Larger volumes than that consumed quickly can cause the patient to aspirate which means droplets go into the lungs.

Over 40 years ago, I was a resident physician assigned for a month to a Pediatric Emergency Department. In those days there were no poison control centers manned by poison experts. It was us! We would get a call about a poisoning and we would try to find the best advice from books or microfiche.

A doctor called and said his patient took several ounces of bleach. I checked the microfilm and found that this was a low-level poison. I advised the doctor to have the patient drink water to dilute it.

Then I had a flash of brilliant insight.

I said, "Doctor, your patient's real problem may be psychiatric"

That's when the doctor said, "Oh, my patient is a dog, I'm a vet."

At that point, I wished him good luck and advised I had human patients to attend.

The Trillion Dollar Bandwagon: A Brief History of Fixing Blocked Coronary Arteries

Let's look at the example of the repair of blocked coronary arteries. Doesn't everybody know fixing blocked arteries is a great thing?

Certainly, one remarkable advance in medical science has been Coronary Artery Bypass Grafting (CABG). For the reader unfamiliar with the purpose of coronary arteries: these are the blood supply to the heart muscle. If these pipes get badly blocked you get chest pain, rhythm disturbances, or shortness of breath and, if a clot forms inside a coronary artery, a heart attack. With a bypass, the surgeon inserts a vein taken from the patient's leg in such a way that the blood can flow around or bypass the blockage. Then fresh blood can get to the heart muscle.

In 1973, when I was in medical school starting my clinical rotations, we thought fixing blocked coronary arteries was something fantastic. The first case had been done in 1960 but it did not become popular then. True, the patient having this new surgical procedure faced an alarming risk of potentially fatal complications. This was new and new stuff is riskier. Yet, we were amazed by the concept. Surgeons were fixing blocked arteries on the surface of the heart!

A few years later as CABG came into wider use, fellowship training programs were developed specifically to train cardiac surgeons. That was clearly better than the on-the-job CABG training available to vascular surgeons up to that point. Specialized training made a big difference in the results. Improved techniques of cardiac anesthesia and smarter post-operative care proved to be of further benefit. The rate of complications fell sharply from the early days. To those of us in medical practice, as well as the general public, bypasses seemed even more marvelous than they had at first.

Every hospital had to have its heart surgery program, and did those programs ever bring in the money! Hospitals competed for star surgeons. For many hospitals, the reputation of the institution itself depended on the reputation of the cardiac surgery program. It seemed as though an endless supply of patients were lined up for these procedures.

I'm not sure how many doctors considered whether the CABG procedures were done on the right patients or whether they were done too often. The focus was on the blockages more than on the patient. Does it always help to fix a blockage? It seemed obvious. Yes, of course! Perhaps doubts came up when our patient or our friend was one of the 1% who died from the procedure. This situation was especially sad if the patient had presented with no symptoms.

How did that happen? Doctors figured that doing a cardiac stress or treadmill test might be good for anybody at a certain age, and sure enough some patients without symptoms "failed" the treadmill test and were taken to the cath lab and found to have some coronary artery blockages. Then they had surgery and faced that 1% mortality rate from the surgery.

Come again? Someone who had no complaints went in for a treadmill test and a few weeks later they died after bypass surgery?

But when someone died, we consoled ourselves by thinking, "Look at all the patients we saved!"

Next, coronary artery stents were invented and quickly came into wide use. You didn't have to split the sternum and spread the ribs to reach the heart and then implant a vein over a blocked artery. You could insert a stent, a springy metal coil, thru an artery via a tube called a catheter. The stent was opened at the proper spot and smashed the cholesterol blockage out of the way, which opened the partial blockage. Stents, we thought, must be better because they were quicker, less expensive, and not painful during recovery. With stents, there was no need to "crack" the sternum. Now we could fix even more patients with blocked arteries. And there were a lot of arteries out there to be fixed!

More People Jump On the Bandwagon. Come On! Won't You Fix My Blocked Arteries?

Patients knew heart attacks were the number one killer. The owner of a blocked coronary artery wanted it repaired. People who feared they had a blocked coronary artery had tests done to see if they had that problem. Why wait for symptoms? More treadmill tests lead to more heart catheterizations. The cardiologists and surgeons were happy to provide a service that seemed to be justified by common sense. If it's completely or even mostly blocked, fix it!

If someone suddenly died of a heart attack people would say, "Why didn't his doctor have him run a routine treadmill test so they could have saved him?" It is now known that most heart attacks are the result of a clot forming on a partly blocked coronary artery. In that situation, the partly blocked artery often won't lead to an abnormal treadmill test. But at that time, people thought the blockages in the arteries just got worse year after year until "Bingo!" you had a heart attack.

I recall a malpractice case I read about in a medical journal. The patient was only in his early 40s but he had all the risk factors. He was obese, the obesity around the middle led to type 2 diabetes, he smoked, he was inactive, he had high cholesterol, and he had a bad family history. This case happened before the recognition of the "Metabolic Syndrome" which is the association of diabetes, heart attack, and stroke with central obesity, elevated cholesterol, elevated triglycerides, hypertension, and type 2 diabetes. This 40-year-old man had a physical with good or only slightly elevated numbers except for his weight. A few months later he suddenly died of a heart attack.

The family sued the doctor and won. Should the patient have lost weight? Taken cholesterol medication? Developed an exercise program? Those considerations were not addressed by the court. The conclusion: the doctor should have predicted his high-risk status and ordered a treadmill test.

Would a treadmill have been positive? Would a bypass have been recommended? Would that have stopped that 40-year-old man from dying?

You see, the idea that even patients without symptoms would be helped by stents or bypasses was just a theory, a hypothesis, a hunch. It might have been true, or not. The answer to that question should have been demonstrated by a number of good research studies *before* it become a part of routine practice. Did we consider it might have been just a promising theory that would turn out to be wrong?

Many standard medical practices are based on promising ideas that have yet to be proven to be right.☼

For years and years a great number of doctors worked under this hypothesis: fixing any badly blocked coronary artery was good for the patient. The skeptics did not go for it.

Another hypothesis came around. Some academic researchers COMPARED regions of the country where a lot of these procedures were done, where they had big medical centers and lots of trained cardiac proceduralists AGAINST places where fewer procedures were done, such as states with fewer surgery programs. Surprise! The death rates from heart disease were the same.

Shouldn't the places with bigger bypass and stent programs have lower numbers or rates of cardiac death?

The alternate hypothesis (hunch) to explain this failure to show a difference was that in most cases, these procedures only help patients get rid of chest symptoms. On average, they don't help patients live longer.

I knew of this hypothesis since about 1999 because I listened to "conservative" cardiologists. But the action-oriented cardiologists advised doing things like stents or bypasses to blocked coronary arteries, and that's what people believed was best. I started to harbor doubts about the cardiologists who did not present the alternative choice to the patients - the choice to not fix it now.

So here's what's behind this curtain: bypassing or stenting a blocked coronary artery helps when symptoms like exertional chest pain are the problem. When we fix bad-looking arteries in patients without symptoms, these procedures may be more dangerous than helpful.

There's one more thing to think about. Let's say the average bypass lasts 12 years. In other words, the bypass grafts can get blockages too. Let's imagine two patients with mild angina. They both have a heart cath and cardiologists find some blockages in the coronary arteries that explain the exertional symptoms (chest pain or shortness of breath with exertion). Both these patients have a life expectancy of 15 years otherwise. Patient #1 gets a bypass now and 12 years later needs a repeat bypass procedure. The other patient waits 5 years for the first bypass and needs a second procedure, not 12 years but 17 years later. But he was only going to live another 15 years, so he only faced the trauma and risks of the bypass procedure once. Did I mention that repeat bypass surgery is more dangerous? If you get your bypass when your symptoms were very mild, you may need a second surgery later if you were young enough. If you wait, you're better off because you come to your end, whenever that was supposed to be, without the second surgery.

More studies are being published. It's still a complex issue but, in general, the better idea seems to be, when the blockages cause no symptoms or only mild symptoms, just wait. In 2019 a new study was publicized. It concluded that just as many patients survived blocked coronary arteries with pills compared with procedures to open or bypass the blockages. As reported in the NY Times:

> "This is far from the first study to suggest that stents and bypass are overused. But previous results have not deterred doctors, who have called earlier research on the subject inconclusive and the design of the trials flawed." Another quote "Stenting and bypass procedures, however, did help some patients with intractable chest pain, called angina."
> NY Times: November 16, 2019.

https://www.nytimes.com/2019/11/16/health/heart-disease-stents-bypass.html

Patient Don't Understand This Fact About the Coronary Circulation

To me it seemed like some surgeons, seeing a severely blocked coronary artery, acted like the knight in shining armor finding a damsel in distress. Ride in there and rescue her. There's not a moment to lose before the dragon shows up.

But the heart has circulation that you don't appreciate on the images of the coronary arteries taken during a heart cath. That section of heart muscle that seems like it would not get enough fresh blood from that one badly blocked artery may be getting enough from the other coronary arteries. You see, the coronary arteries originate in the upper part of the heart, but in the lower part of the heart all the major arterial branches come together. The Left Anterior Descending (LAD) artery runs over the front of the left ventricle. When the LAD is blocked, some blood gets to its part of the heart via the Circumflex artery, which goes around the back of the left ventricle and heads towards the bottom of the heart (which is oddly called the apex), and then sends tiny branches around to the front. If that description is too obtuse, I'll simplify: **the heart has its own backup blood supply system.**

The studies show that fixing blockages in patients without significant symptoms does not save lives. Maybe that's because our hearts have this backup system. It's OK to jump off the bandwagon, to refuse the procedures in these cases.

Although fixing any badly blocked artery became a common practice, it was always just a theory that these procedures helped everyone. Now we realize it is not a necessary thing to do for a patient without bad symptoms.

This new truth is not universally accepted even today. We believed in the logic of our old theory and when data came in that contradicted that theory many doctors and patients ignored it.

In other words: the data challenging the conventional wisdom was ignored by many because it challenged conventional wisdom.☼

Memory Past and Future: Memory of Mistakes

I observed in anxious and depressed patients a great deal of worrying about things in the past. I would tell my patients it is hard to do a good job driving forward if you keep your eye on the rearview mirror. Think about that.

Certainly, we have to learn from the past. As I mentioned in another essay, Oscar Wilde said, "Experience is merely the name men give to their mistakes."

So when we speak of someone with a lot of experience, do we mean someone who's made a lot of mistakes?

I'd like to see a job posting with that in mind. Instead of listing, "Five years of experience required," it would say, "We require five years of making mistakes."

I would say you really can't call it "experience" unless you have learned from those mistakes and then you apply those lessons to future decision-making.

But some people are dominated by their past memories and think about them all the time. If what you did could have been done better or differently, you should just figure out if there is some lesson for the future in your mistake and then move on.

Memory In Anxiety, Depression, and PTSD

I don't pretend at all to understand posttraumatic stress disorder, but I wonder if one part of the disorder is not being able to let go of memories that are better to let fade away.

Among the elements in the Diagnostic and Statistic Manual defining posttraumatic stress disorder are "intrusive thoughts" and "flashbacks." I observed that many patients with anxiety and depression exhibited difficulty forgetting. Patients with these disorders have trouble falling asleep because their minds keep playing the same thoughts over and over again. It's a very common symptom.

The healthy brain can dismiss these memories.

The word "memory" is useful to describe the function. Specifically, we know there is RECALL memory in which you can think of something when you need it, and there is RECOGNITION memory, which means you don't remember it until you see a prompt, a reminder. The nice thing about multiple-choice tests in school is they allow you to use your recognition memory in addition to your recall memory.

I went to college in Princeton, New Jersey, not far from Trenton, the capital. I would advise my patients that Trenton is the capital of New Jersey. "Can you memorize that?"

That's easy enough. Then I would say, "Okay, can you just please forget that Trenton is the capital of New Jersey?" Of course, the answer was no. Forgetting things is not a skill we have.

Or is it? Well, it does happen, we do forget things. The forgetting just happens in the background. It can't happen when we're paying attention. You can't say, "I choose to forget what I had for breakfast." But it may just get forgotten when you are busy fixing dinner.

Westworld Robots Had Digital Memory

In the award-winning HBO series Westworld, well-heeled tourists vacationed in a fictional Western land populated by very human-like robots or androids. Some of the robots were programmed to take the role of bad guys. The tourists, mostly men who were wannabe gunslingers, could shoot and otherwise abuse the android actors who then "died." That night the bloodied robots were carted back to the robot repair building where they were patched up, memory wiped, and reprogrammed.

Many of the female robots served as sex objects for the tourists. They were romanced or raped and received every type of violence perpetrated against women. After that, back to the repairmen, memory wiped, reprogrammed.

But there was a defect in the design of the androids' artificial memories. Deeply buried memories of being killed or abused persisted after the memory wipes. The psychological trauma survived in hidden areas of their memory banks.

Sometimes these robots had flashbacks. They had been killed or raped or both hundreds of times and these memories would replay at random times. The robots had no control over when or whether these memories replayed. And because the memories were digital, they were perfect copies. All at once, a digital memory would be replayed in the mind of a robot just as we could replay a DVR of a TV show. And the memories were seen in the robot mind as clearly as in real life.

In other words, robots couldn't tell flashbacks from real life; it looked the same to them when their brains replayed them. From their viewpoint they were truly back in the past, not just remembering it but actually being there.

The effect of replaying all these horrible memories over and over: the robots turned against the humans.

As a doctor, I probably looked at the show a little differently than other people. I realized the good thing about the way our brains work is that we can tell that memory is not real life. Memories are fuzzy. Memories are incomplete. We should really take comfort from that.

If you have a condition that causes you to replay your bad memories and over, get help for that. Counseling and/or medication may help.

Memory Interfering With Sleep

Sometimes when you're falling asleep and your brain starts replaying the same thought over and over again, the only thing you can do is find something else to keep your brain busy.

I must mention that if this is happening too often, see your doctor. It could be a symptom of severe anxiety or depression. Medication or counseling might help you.

If this happens to me when I'm trying to fall asleep, I try counting backward. Counting sheep never made sense to me. I'll pick a number under 1000 like 775 and then start counting backward. I tell myself if I get to 600, I'll get up out of bed and do something. Sometimes I don't just say the number to myself, I force myself to picture the number on a mailbox.

Sometimes the numbers are black, sometimes blue, sometimes red, sometimes raised, and sometimes reflective, but they are always different from one number to the next. I can keep my brain really busy doing this.

Sometimes I count backward by 1,2,3 etc. steps. It's complicated and hard to describe. I'll start with something like 801. 801 minus 1 is 800. 800 minus 2 in 798. 798 minus 3 is 795. You see I'm subtracting one more each time. 795 minus 4 is 791. 791 minus 5 in 786. 786 minus 6 is 780. Got the idea? That exercise really drives the other thoughts away.

Sometimes, if I'm not into numbers, I can think about how I make coffee. I know the drill; I do it the same every time. Measure out the beans, put them in the grinder, form the paper filter, and place the filter in the filter holder. Put the ground beans in the a small bowl. Blow out the grinder with compressed air in a can. Weigh the exact amount of water that will fill my cup. Boil the water in the microwave. Insert the digital thermometer and stir. Watch the temperature as it falls. At just below 203 degrees add the coffee grinds and stir. Put the filter holder and filter onto the cup. Wait five minutes. Pour the mixture into the filter and let it run through... you have the idea. It's a series of tasks that I always do the same way every day and the exercise of thinking through each step keeps my brain occupied. Whoops...I just revealed I don't use a coffee maker when making a single cup. When all those unnecessary memories are pushed away by coffee-making thoughts, then sleep might come.

Everyone Has to Die But I Had Hoped They Might Make An Exception in My Case

New trees can get started in the forest only after the old trees fall over. Then sunlight can reach the young plants on the forest floor. In the forest, death is necessary for new life.

When I was in junior high school I began a fascination with science fiction. This time was well after Buck Rogers and well before Star Wars. I don't think many students in our school were reading from the science fiction section in the school library. I found some stories in those books were surprisingly racy, especially by the standards of the early 60s which were more like the 50s. They say the real 60's didn't happen until the Beatles. I recall one story I read about a planet that had a big war. Only one man survived but millions of women were looking for a partner. The surviving man had to sleep with a different woman each night to keep humankind going. My 12-year-old self thought, "That would be very tiring!"

I remember another story about a young couple who lived in a future where doctors had conquered all illnesses. People lived hundreds of years. The couple wanted to get married but they couldn't afford a place to live. Because people weren't dying as much, the population grew and grew and housing prices skyrocketed. The couple were each still living with their parents who in turn were living with their parents were still living with their parents who were still living with their parents.

The "young" couple in question were in their 80s.

So in this story, the absence of death messed up the housing supply.

As a doctor, you must accept the necessity of death at an earlier stage of life than others. We all know we are all going to die. We are going to leave this body behind. This truth doesn't strike you when you are young in most other professions.

I remember seeing a deceased person's body for the first time. I was 19. I had a job as a morgue attendant in the Hamilton County Ohio Coroner's Office after my sophomore year of college. I saw a lot of deceased bodies. I thought that dead people looked like wax museum manikins, except for the lack of pink in their color. I thought to myself, when you die you become a wax museum figure.

That thought made it easier when we did the autopsy on that body. I learned the job quickly. Part of my job was to open the skull and remove the brain for the pathologist. The technique was such that the incision was easily hidden later from the mourners at the funeral parlor.

In those days there was no synthetic growth hormone, so in that less litigious age, without any permission and without testing for hepatitis B, etc. we would take the pituitary gland. You had to remove the brain first and then open the *sella turcica*, a bony depression in the base of the skull, and there was the pituitary gland, the size of a large pea. We put the glands in a jar. They were sent to companies that extracted and sold the growth hormone they contained for the benefit of children with growth hormone deficiency.

It was nice to think the dead were helping the living, even if no one else knew.

The head morgue attendant was an older fellow. He told me he would never fly in an airplane. He said, "When you're going to go, you're going to go. But in an airplane, if the pilot is going to go, you're going to go too. I don't think he understood the role of the copilot.

People ask me, "How do you remember all this stuff." I say, "How can you forget it?"

54

Five days before his death, the author William Saroyan wrote, "Everybody has to die but I always believed an exception would be made in my case."

I can sympathize with his attitude. I think a lot of us have the same idea.

The Concept of Medical Reversal and Replacement

Medical care gradually changes. Vinay Prasad MD and Adam Cifu, MD wrote a book about "Medical Reversals" in 2015.

Medical reversal occurs when a new clinical trial — superior to earlier scientific trials by virtue of better design, placebo controls, size, or measures of outcome — contradicts current clinical practice.

Replacement is the related change in practice that should follow when the new way replaces the old.

Two problems occur.

(1) Some new approaches are adopted too quickly before definitive studies (which can take years and years) have been performed. Later that new approach that looked so promising is withdrawn after newer data comes out. That's called another reversal.

(2) Some old ways of treatment need to be replaced but the new ways are not implemented into widespread use even after the new definitive studies have been publicized.

The authors explain that new and better, new treatments will replace older, less effective treatments over time. They give the example that biting on a bullet during surgery has been replaced by anesthesia.

In modern medicine, when critical new evidence is published, it can take decades for new tests or treatment approaches to replace popular old ones. Doctors often actively fight them. This sounds surprising, doesn't it?

Let's consider this quotation from Upton Sinclair. You probably learned about him in high school. He was famous for writing his book about the meat processing industry, The Jungle, in 1906. He revealed that the meat used in processing plants was often rotten and diseased. The book was very popular and within the year, Congress passed the Pure Food and Drug Act and the Meat Inspection Act, which were signed into law by President Teddy Roosevelt. The new laws were enforced by the Bureau of Chemistry within the Department of Agriculture which became the FDA in 1930.

Upton Sinclair wrote:

It is difficult to get a man to understand something when his salary depends upon his not understanding it.

Consider three examples Prasad and Cifu provide.

Old idea: mammography for women in their 40s is valuable, it saves lives. New idea: studies showed mammography for women in their 40s is largely ineffective as far as saving lives.

Whose salary depends upon not understanding the new evidence?:

Among others, radiologists who read mammograms, hospitals who invested in expensive machines, manufacturers who make mammography machines, doctors who treat cancer, mammography centers, and manufacturers of chemotherapy drugs.

Old idea: Prostate cancer screening with rectal exam and/or PSA testing saves lives. PSA testing is an example of something that gained great popular use before complete testing had been finished. I mean we should have waited for studies that showed that the benefit of the screening was greater than the harms.

New idea: New studies showed far more harm than good results from such screening. Only one in 50 men treated for prostate cancer found by screening this way are actually saved from dying. PSA screening only saves one in 1400 men tested by screening after 13 years. Many tested are found to have cancer. They get treated and then develop permanent side effects despite the treatment not helping them live longer. The latest guideline tells us from age 55 to 69 the decision to screen should be individualized based on risk factors and patient values pertaining to risk and benefit.

What does "patient values" mean? It could mean how would you answer this question: "Suppose you had the PSA test and it were positive, and then you had a biopsy and it was positive for cancer and you then found yourself next in a room with 50 men who like you had been found to have prostate cancer by screening and they told all 50 of you that with radical prostatectomy or radiation therapy one person in the room might live who would otherwise die from the cancer, but that more than half of you who weren't helped would have loss of erection or some loss of bladder control. Would you leave the room or stay for the surgery or other treatments?" **If you would not stay in the room, why have the PSA test in the first place?**☼

Whose "salary depends upon" not understanding the new evidence?: Among others, urologists, hospital administrators, cancer doctors, manufacturers of robotic surgery devices, radiation therapists and treatment centers, and chemotherapy manufacturers.

Old idea: Any coronary artery with a significant blockage should be stented, to prevent heart attacks and extend life.

New idea: Studies show for a limited number of years, stents will relieve chest pain caused by exertion, but stents do not prolong life or prevent heart attacks.

Whose "salary depends upon" not understanding the new evidence?: Among others, Cardiologists who specialize in placing stents, hospital administrators, and manufacturers of stents.

Patients need to be aware that medical practice changes slowly at times even among those whose "salary does not depend upon" not understanding the new evidence. Why? **Because doctors feel most comfortable practicing the way other doctors practice even if conventional ways of practice should be abandoned.**☼

"Bob, No Number of Signed Releases Will Prevent You From Being Sued"

I remember when I was Chief of Family Medicine at my hospital. At that time it seemed screening for prostate cancer with the PSA blood test had become the routine. Never before had so many cancers of the prostate been discovered! Never before had so many men been subjected to radical prostatectomy! Never before had so many Family Doctors and urologists basked in the glow of grateful patients who declared their lives had been saved by early detection! Never before were so many post-prostatectomy patients suffering from urinary incontinence or erectile dysfunction!

A paper had been published in the Journal of Family Practice that proposed that a PSA should never be performed on a patient without a release being signed. The subtitle of the article was "truth in advertising." The release would warn the patient that the PSA had not been proven to save lives yet but was known to result in a lot of harm (pain, impotence, needle biopsies through the rectum, and side effects of surgery, radiation, and chemotherapy). One author, Richard G Roberts, MD was both an attorney and a Family Doctor. His paper was published before the studies were completed: the studies that showed that PSA screening was either not effective or minimally effective at saving lives.

Those studies should have been completed first before the PSA screening had been put into widespread use

I read the article and was convinced Dr. Roberts and his colleagues were on to something. After all, we had learned in medical school that autopsy studies showed many older men had small prostate cancers, never knew it, and died of other things without finding out. How many men had some prostate cancer? About 40% by age 40. About 70% of men by age 70.

I asked myself: Why in the world did we want to test for all those cancers? Why treat so many?

Being Chief, I ran the monthly Family Practice meetings. I tried to keep the doctors informed about any issue that could affect the care delivered at the hospital. At a meeting in early 1994, I brought up the subject of the article. "Maybe we should warn men that this new and very popular PSA test might do more harm than good. The response of the doctors in my department was instantaneous and unanimous. "Bob," one doctor said, "If you have a patient who dies of prostate cancer and you didn't do a PSA, you are going to be sued for malpractice. No number of signed releases will prevent that."

My doctors did not profit from PSA testing. They just sensed that everyone did it and the best course was to practice the way everyone else did.

Regardless, from that time onward, I doggedly refused to order a screening PSA without giving the patient a careful explanation of the other side of the controversy - whether it was good to screen. Then I left it up to the patient. That discussion always put me behind schedule, but I always thought to myself "Screw the schedule."

Years later, Richard Ablin, Ph.D., the researcher who discovered the science behind the PSA test but did not profit from it, wrote a book called, The Great Prostate Hoax: How Big Medicine Hijacked the PSA Test and Caused a Public Health Disaster. I guess you can tell which side he was on.

In the early 1990s, we thought the answer to whether to screen with the PSA would be forthcoming within the next decade. The long-term trials had begun but the results were far off. Not until 2009 did we get the results of two long-awaited long-term studies. The European (ERSPC) and the American (PLCO) trial.

The American study showed no benefit to the PSA test as screening. The European one showed minimal benefit. Specifically for every 1000 men screened, 0.7 deaths were prevented. That is one life saved for every 1410 men screened. To save this one life, 49 men had to be treated for prostate cancer. That was the European study.

In 2018 the results of another trial were released. This was the largest-ever trial of PSA testing in men over age 50, a study involving 400,000 men. It showed that after ten years of follow-up, there was no difference in the number of deaths from Prostate cancer between those who were screened and those who were not. This study was called, "Effect of a Low-Intensity PSA-Based Screening Intervention on Prostate Cancer Mortality: The CAP Randomized Clinical Trial." JAMA, March 6, 2018.

Since then other studies have shown slightly more benefit of PSA screening in selected patients.

What about the old way of checking for cancer of the prostate, the digital rectal exam (DRE)? That's not a test for early prostate cancer. If the doctor can feel it, it's already advanced. DRE is good to evaluate the man with symptoms.

This topic is likely to change over time. To get the latest, look up the recommendations of the United States Preventative Services Taskforce. I could give you the URL, but I want you to explore this website and be properly amazed at the thoroughness of their research. Their work is impressive and their bias is in favor of evidence. They don't make recommendations based on "that's the way everyone practices."

Screening For Colon Cancer

This might be a more interesting topic because it applies to everyone once you get older, not just men. Screening for colon cancer is not controversial. The United States Preventive Services Task Force, or USPSTF, recommends screening starting at age 45 and strongly recommends screening at ages 50 to 75. For people over 75 the benefit is much smaller and might not be worth it.

Before colonoscopy was standard, I was doing sigmoidoscopy in my office. That's like colonoscopy but you one go up 60 inches and don't use anesthesia. I "scoped" about 200 people. I found a lot of polyps and those patients then went for colonoscopies. I found only two cancerous polyps.

One patient with a malignant polyp was a man of about 50. He had it removed. He complained endlessly about the bother of the whole thing and the time he lost from work. He never thanked me for likely saving his life. Maybe he thanked me so quietly I didn't hear him. That was OK. I knew.

The other person with a cancerous tumor was a lady with severe chronic lung disease. I found her polyp and referred her to a specialist for the removal. After that they wanted to do major surgery to remove a segment of her sigmoid and rectum. She would have a colostomy. I asked her lung doctor, "Is that safe for her?" The lung specialist said, "Not really." I advised against the proposed surgery.

Her lung disease killed her about two years later. The colon cancer never came back.

The idea is to detect polyps. Those are the little bumps inside your colon that grow into cancer and sometimes already contain a bit of cancer when discovered. At this stage the cancer has not spread, we hope.

Ronald Reagan had a colonoscopy just after his reelection. They found cancer in a polyp and it was removed. A few months later, at a press conference, a reporter asked, "Mr. President, how's your cancer?"

Reagan said something like: "What cancer?"

The reporter at first didn't know how to respond. Then he said, "Mr. President, we were told that you had a cancerous polyp removed."

Reagan said, "The polyp had cancer, not me."

A lot of people assume screening means a colonoscopy every ten years. But there are less invasive ways to screen that are nearly as good. ☼

If you don't know, colonoscopy means a doctor puts a tube into your rectum when you are sedated. The tube has a camera on the end. The doctor pushes and pulls and rotates the tube in such a way that it slides up and up and all the way around the colon. It doesn't hurt if they give you enough anesthesia.

The last time I had a colonoscopy, I woke up twice in the middle of the procedure due to discomfort. The pain was very unpleasant but at least it was brief. I wasn't given enough anesthesia.

How sensitive is colonoscopy? "Sensitive" means do we find all the polyps and cancers that are there? You would think that all the polyps 10 mm or large would be readily found, but the colon is oddly curved and polyps can hide among the twists and turns. Only about 89 to 95% of polyps that large are found with the scope.

Other tests involve testing stool samples for blood. The idea is that polyps bleed a bit. High sensitivity stool tests find 50 to 75% of colon cancers. That 89 to 95% colonoscopy sensitivity stat mentioned above was for polyps, whether cancerous or not.

Another test is called a fecal immunochemical test. This test finds 74% of cancers, per the USPSTF.

The leading stool test is called Colo-guard. It measures stool for blood AND cancer DNA. It finds 93% of the cancers but only 43% of the larger polyps.

The good thing about the stool tests is you don't need to take laxatives and enemas to clean out your colon first. The bad thing is, if the test is positive you need a colonoscopy anyway.

Another point about colon cancer that many patients don't know is that low-dose aspirin may lower the risk by 40%. ☼ Aspirin is not recommended for everyone. Aspirin might NOT be a good idea if you have a history of ulcers, are over 70, or have uncontrolled hypertension, but might be a better idea if you have risk factors for colon cancer such as diabetes, obesity, or hypertension. Unfortunately, the full effect of low-dose aspirin in lowering the risk of colon cancer requires ten years of taking it daily.

Screening, Bleeding, and Bidets

Here's something that most patients don't understand about the cost of colonoscopy. Screening means testing people who have no symptoms. The Affordable Care Act made all health insurance companies cover screening for colon cancer at 100%. You would suffer no expense other than the cost of getting to the test or loss of time from work.

If you report a bit of blood from your bottom, it's a different story. ☼ The same test is now called a diagnostic colonoscopy. Not free. If you have a $1000 deductible, you are going to pay $1000 for it, unless you have already met your deductible for the year. Now you might get cleaned out twice: once with the laxatives and enemas for the test and a second time when you pay your deductible.

What to do? If you bleed on the toilet and report it to the doctor, that could save your life. Pay the man! Or...

Here's something I never heard doctors recommend vis-a-vis colon cancer testing. You might save yourself some grief by getting one of those $60 bidet attachments that fit over your toilet bowl. Rather than rub your bottom with toilet paper, which can cause bleeding, you wash with a stream of water: much less chance you will see blood from irritation of those delicate tissues. Also, there would be less risk of developing chronic itching of the anus due to over-vigorously rubbing or from leaving traces of stool behind after using toilet paper. ☼ With the bidet, you need no more rubbing. You only use toilet paper to blot yourself dry.

When you think about it, it's kind of disgusting how we clean our bottoms with paper! If you were to get stool on your hands, like when changing a poopy diaper, you wouldn't just wipe them off with toilet paper, would you?

You might say, "If I see blood on the toilet paper, I know it's just a hemorrhoid." Guess what? Most family doctors after a decade of practice have seen patients who reported blood only on the toilet paper AND had hemorrhoids, but they also had a colon cancer growing ten inches or more up from the hemorrhoids. Here's the rule: hemorrhoids don't immunize you against colon cancer.

One caveat. The most affordable bidets don't heat the water. They just connect to the cold line. If it's winter in the cold climates and someone just flushed before you and if the line is close to an outside wall, you will get a very cold wash down there. Turn the knob carefully. Just wash with a trickle of water Freezing your bottom in the winter is still better than getting the prep for a colonoscopy.

Royalty

When I was in residency training, another resident physician I knew had been moonlighting in the emergency department of the hospital in a nearby town.

My friend made a comment that he disliked working in that ER.

He said, "The people from that town think they are royalty ."

I asked him what he meant by that and he said, "They all want to be treated as if they were somebody special."

One of our faculty members was an older doctor who had lived and practiced in that town for 30 years or more. I'll just call him Dr. Jones.

I was curious about what my faculty mentor would think about my friend's critique of the patients from his town. I relayed what he had said.

Dr. Jones bristled. "Of course they act like royalty. We've been treating them like they were royalty for as long as I can remember."

I found his attitude inspiring. Throughout my career, when I had a difficult new patient who came with an attitude of entitlement or some chip on his shoulder, I didn't let it bother me. I tried to treat him as if he were a member of "royalty" too.

When dealing with such a patient that some would label as "difficult," I might tell the medical student. "Let's think about this patient as if we knew he were the brother of the President of the United States."

About 15 years into my own practice, one of the consultants told me, "You have the nicest patients. How did you get so many nice people to come to you?"

I thought about that. Most of my patients came to me because other patients recommended me. This was in the days before you had to pick your family doctor out of a book

66

of doctors who had signed up to accept the fees and practice stipulations of your insurance company.

It occurred to me that maybe my people just acted nice because they had been treated with respect. You reap what you sow... that sort of thing.

Since You Realize That in Medicine We May Be Slow to Change How We Practice or We May Adopt New Things Before They Are Truly Proven, What's Next? Trust the Doctor Who Is Willing to Answer All Your Questions. But what to ask?

I am going to repeat that last sentence from two chapters back. "The data challenging the conventional wisdom was ignored by many because it challenged conventional wisdom."

Let me acknowledge that research on outcomes is ongoing. It's not finished. It may never be finished. Furthermore, it's impossible to make good decisions today based on research that won't be published until a year or 5 years from now.

But when research already published and confirmed by other studies shows a better way than usual practice, and experts corroborate the conclusions, we doctors are often slow to make changes in our usual practices. The retreat from fixing every significant-looking coronary artery blockage has been slow. It's taking decades for this retreat to take hold.

Bottom line, if you have blocked arteries in your heart but NO SYMPTOMS such as exertional chest pain, pressure, or shortness of breath with exertion, and the interventional cardiologist wants to fix the blockages, you have the option to get another opinion. When the doctor doing the procedure has an opening in his procedure schedule, it may seem like an urgent situation to him, but it isn't urgent for you. Get a second opinion. They may advise you to try medication. Again, this idea applies to patients with no symptoms.

When you are about to have a diagnostic heart cath, they may ask you to sign a consent for a procedure to fix any blockages discovered, "just in case."

"Due to the anesthesia, you will be "out of it" and we cannot get your consent then. Can you sign now?"

If you are the patient who doesn't have symptoms such as chest pressure, pain, or shortness of breath during exercise or emotional stress or if you haven't tried the usual medications first, *don't* sign the consent in advance of the procedure. The question for discussion is whether to have a stent placed. Make that decision with your regular cardiologist after you wake up and give yourself the chance to think over the options and if necessary get another opinion.

Please note: there may be exceptions to this rule like a seriously obstructed left main coronary artery or a 100% blockage of the Left Anterior Descending (LAD) at its beginning, called a "widowmaker" lesion. The left main is a short segment that supplies the LAD and the Circumflex, the two arteries that supply the left ventricle (main pumping muscle). These serious blockages usually cause symptoms, but large blockages in these arteries without symptoms are dangerous regardless. Left main lesions normally need a bypass but hi-grade blockages of the LAD can be stented. These possibilities should be part of the discussion before your initial heart cath.

Were I an asymptomatic patient about to have my coronary arteries catheterized, I'd sign something that said, "We will only place a stent if we find a high-grade LAD blockage; in addition, we may arrange for emergency CABG if you have a high-grade Left Main blockage.

I'm not trying to give you specific advice applying to you as a patient. I am giving advice about choices in general. Your cardiologist may have different rules for the "only stent me if you find this lesion" problem

I started this discussion by saying not to give conventional medicine your unconditional trust. As imperfect as it may be, conventional practice is a lot better than the crap that some kooky charlatans invent and offer for sale on the internet. But you still need a big touch of skepticism with the conventional.

Sometimes you need to talk with the doctor you know well and trust, like your family doctor, to find out which questions to ask the specialist.

Examples of some very pointed questions:

Doctor, I understand your reasons for doing this procedure but do studies show that performing this procedure *now* is better than waiting until later?

"Well, in my opinion..."

Doctor, I didn't make my question clear. When I said, "do studies show?" I was not asking your personal opinion on that last point.

Doctor, I read about a concept called the "Number Needed to Treat" I realize surgery doesn't always work and medicine is not an exact science but roughly how many of these procedures must be done before one patient in my situation is helped?

Doctor, how many deaths are expected per 100 procedures like the one you are proposing?

Doctor, you told me of the possible complications, but for every 100 procedures how many patients develop long-lasting side effects or other issues as a result of this procedure?

Doctor, how many procedures of this type have you personally performed?

Doctor are there any controversies about this procedure? Are there reports or editorials in the medical literature that suggest this procedure is less worthwhile than believed or that it should be done less often?

Asking tough questions might prompt your doctor to think harder for you.

Trust your doctor after you have had your questions answered.

My Best Worst Teacher

In residency training we learn to think, we learn to do and we fashion the type of doctor we will become. You learn a lot from great doctors. Unexpectedly, I learned a lot from one of the worst doctors I'd ever met. He's been gone for a long time. That man is not the subject here. My topic is how he treated patients during the month I spent with him.

During residency, young doctors get assigned to different attending physicians, or for short, "attendings." I was a first-year resident, traditionally called an "intern." This unforgettable attending moved through rounds with the speed of lightning. He could round on eight patients in an hour. One of the ways he kept on schedule was by not answering complicated questions.

On the first day of the rotation, we had an 80-year-old lady who had suffered a heart attack and was just out of the intensive care unit. Her heart had developed a serious rhythm disturbance and the Coronary Care Unit doctors had needed to apply defibrillator paddles to deliver an electric shock to the heart.

But for some technical reason having to do with how the round paddles were applied during the crisis, she suffered a crescent-shaped first-degree burn right in the middle of her chest. A first-degree burn, just redness, is a minor burn.

It was the first day of the month, the first day we had rounded with this attending physician. Before going into the room he said, "If the old lady asks about the burn on her chest don't answer the question, I don't want to get into all that, it will take forever to explain, it will get us behind and it will get her too worried."

Sure enough, as soon as the attending asked "How are you doing?" she asked, "Doctor, what's this on my chest?"

He said, "We'll talk about that tomorrow."

When we were out in the hallway racing to the next patient, he assured us that she would surely forget her question by the next day.

But the next morning she asked again and once again he promised he would explain the oddly-shaped red mark on her chest the following day.

And on the third day, she had still not forgotten. She said, "Doctor, I insist you tell me about this red mark on my chest."

At that point, he simply laughed, "Oh that? The guy who did that doesn't work at this garage anymore."

She burst into laughter as did the resident and I. There were no more questions.

I'm pretty sure she already knew what had happened. She was a lot smarter than he gave her credit for. I think she wanted to hear it from him and to know more about why she'd been shocked. Patients often understand more than we doctors think.

71

Five Key Qualities of This Teacher

This doctor was one of my most important teachers! There were at least five personality traits he exhibited that I resolved NEVER to imitate.

1 Lack of respect for the patient,

2 Prioritizing his own time schedule over the patient's welfare,

3 Lack of compassion,

4 Not listening to the patient, and

5 Considering only the first possibility that came to mind rather than multiple possibilities.

On the positive side, I did learn from him that it was OK to joke with a patient. If done well, the patients responded well to humor.

Sometimes we need to go beyond the usual formal tone of explaining things to patients, as long as we remain respectful. If my attending teacher had cracked the joke about the mechanic no longer working in this garage and got the expected laugh, he could have followed up with, "You had a funny rhythm that was best treated with a jolt of electricity. The treatment worked, but the device caused a minor burn that should heal well without treatment." The laughter is the reassurance that the situation is not worth getting stressed over.

But Dr. X was, too often, not respectful. We had a young woman who was in a sad pickle. She wanted to get pregnant. But for a few years, she had suffered repeated blood clots in her legs. Some of those clots traveled to her lungs in the form of potentially life-threatening pulmonary emboli. Her treatment with lifelong anticoagulants caused excessive menstrual bleeding. She became severely anemic several times and needed transfusions. The bleeding was so bad that the iron therapy and the transfusions were not keeping up with the blood loss. The usual ways of controlling her problem simply did not work.

We consulted the gynecology service. Their proposed solution to this situation was a hysterectomy. Ouch: She had not yet had children. She still wanted to have children.

On the day we were planning to discuss the options with her, our attending paused our rounding group a few doors away from her room. He said, "Nobody talk, let me explain this to her."

We entered the room and he said, "I have good news and bad news. The bad news is the gynecologist recommends removing your uterus, but the good news is we can remove the baby bassinet without losing the playpen!"

It was a painful moment for me to watch her reaction. She immediately understood the analogy of sex and pregnancy to baby furniture and began crying her eyes out. My attending did a 180-degree turn and we left the room. I wasn't sure if she was crying because of the future hysterectomy or because of his unfeeling way of communicating.

From what planet did this man arrive? In what worldview does the ability to enjoy sex after a hysterectomy replace the blessing of having a baby?

So I learned that humor may be OK at times but respect for the patient comes first. Turn on the empathy machine before plugging in the humor machine.

Another patient had been admitted with a host of seemingly unrelated complaints. A series of blood tests, scans, and consultations were ordered and performed. Nowadays, the workup would have been done as an outpatient and taken two months to complete, but in those days the insurance companies had not learned to regulate doctors so well.

All the tests came back normal. The attending charged into the room during rounds and announced, "Good news, you can go home, your tests were normal."

That patient looked up and said, "But doctor, what's causing my headache, my back pain, and my stomach problems?

The attending didn't miss a beat. "Oh yeah, you should probably see a psychiatrist for all that but I wouldn't if I were you, they usually can't help people."

I am not kidding, this actually happened.

Principle #1 to not emulate: Lack of respect for the patient,

Principle #3 not to emulate: Lack of compassion,

Think Beyond the First Potential Diagnosis

In another case we had was a lady in her 50s who had the bad luck to have had a thyroid removal surgery that was not done correctly. The skilled surgeon is careful to leave behind at least one of the parathyroid glands. If they don't leave one behind, the patient suffers a deficiency of parathyroid gland hormone, which, unlike thyroid replacement medicine, is not available in pill form. With very experienced surgeons it rarely happens, but in this case, she had been left with no parathyroid function.

Without parathyroid hormone, the blood calcium falls to seriously low levels. This attending, my worst teacher, would admit her every few weeks to give her IV calcium for a few days. Every day he saw her in hospital it was like "CHING" the sound a cash register makes. In and out, one more fee charged.

During the month I was assigned to his service, she was admitted again for IV calcium. I am sure at least a dozen or more young doctors a year got to know this nice lady because interns and residents rotated through this doctor's service every month and she came in all the time.

She was what they called an "easy admission." All we had to do, I was told, was talk to her a little, find out if anything different were going on, and copy all the documentation from the last admission except for anything that might have changed. You have to make up time on the easy cases to save time for the hard ones, right?

But on this admission, something new was happening. She had an upset stomach. The resident prescribed Maalox which contains magnesium hydroxide. Tagamet, the first modern acid-suppressor medication, had not been released by the FDA.

But during our usual light-speed rounds, I came up with a new idea. I asked the attending why we couldn't use calcium carbonate as the antacid instead of magnesium hydroxide. Maybe that would help the chronically low calcium problem, or so I hypothesized. Calcium carbonate was rarely used; everybody prescribed magnesium hydroxide. He said "good idea" and handed the chart to the resident who changed the Maalox two TBS four times a day to Calcium Carbonate but left the dose the same: eight TBS per day. I did not see the order until later, but Calcium carbonate should have been dosed at 1 *teaspoon* four times a day. Since there are three teaspoons in one tablespoon, what she received was six times the recommended dose. She went home on the calcium carbonate at that dose.

A week later she came in with "a stroke." She was groggy and her speech was distorted. CT scans of the head were a brand new thing, the scanners were quite slow and you had to wait until the machine was free, which sometimes took over a day. So on rounds, she had not yet had the brain CT to prove that "stroke." I was the lowly intern on the team, but I spoke up anyway. "While we're waiting on the CT scan, let's check her calcium. High calcium can make you look like this."

The attending laughed and reminded me her problem was low calcium, not high. But we ordered the calcium anyway and it came back three points over the upper normal limits. We stopped the large dose of calcium and hydrated her which lowered her blood calcium and in two days she was speaking clearly and had lost the dazed look. Not only that, but she had a normal calcium. She had not had a stroke after all. We sent her home with a much lower dose of calcium carbonate. Her doctor was able to adjust things as an outpatient so she never needed to come back to the hospital for IV calcium treatments after that, or so I was told.

Principle #5 to not emulate: Considering only the first possibility that comes to mind rather taking the time to consider other possibilities.

I Am No Genius.

Now don't think the point of the last story is that I am some kind of genius doctor. I'm not. Everybody has their brilliant days and their dumb days. But in medicine, each case is different. You need to give your brain a little time to remember the important factors that might make all the difference to the patient.

Now if you spend twice as much time counseling the patient or considering the less common possibilities, the remuneration is about 1.5 times as much. Twice the time, only about 1.5 times the allowed fee. So that is a disincentive to sit and think with the patient.

Now I read there is a proposal by the government to change the fee schedule so that visits of medium to high complexity and very high complexity are all paid the same as short visits. That will result in a strong disincentive to the doctors who have been willing to pause and think.

In medicine, the common possibilities are called horses and the rare ones are called zebras. We are taught that a reasonable person, dozing under the shade of a tree in a pasture in most parts of the world, who is awakened by the sound of hoofbeats behind her, would think of horses before considering zebras. But for speedy doctor X, it could be said: "Differential diagnosis: one horse, zero zebras."

Why was Doctor X one of my best teachers? You learn from your own mistakes, but a much better way is to learn from the mistakes of the people around you.

I want to be respectful to my teachers. Maybe I experienced this doctor during his worst month. That must be it.

"Bob, There's Nothing I Can Do."

A surgical specialist in our town was very busy but you could always get a patient to see him for a minor outpatient procedure; for the others in his specialty, it took weeks. By reputation, he was wealthy from his practice.

When I was in junior high school, I had classmates who were the offspring of doctors. Based on where they lived, I thought their dads might have made twice what mine made. I don't think I was far off. But now we have specialists who make ten or twenty times what average people make. What a world!

I had a patient with diabetes who had developed an infected sebaceous cyst. The infection was early, the cyst was just starting to become pink and tender. I did not like the way it looked because in diabetes infected cysts can go wrong quickly. They start to swell and make a ton of pus.

Because he was very good at performing this type of minor surgical procedure in the office I made the referral to this surgeon. I could get her in right away.

In those days, as it is today in Ohio if you sent Medicare a claim, you had to accept the assignment from Medicare. You could charge whatever you liked, let's say $350, but when the Medicare Explanation of Benefits statement arrived, it might tell you the doctor had to accept $75 for that procedure. The dollar amounts may seem small because this was years ago.

By the way, the people in this and all my stories are disguised.

There was an exception to the assignment requirement. If the procedure was cosmetic, it was deemed "not covered" by Medicare and the doctor could charge and collect whatever he wanted. The doctor could easily manipulate the system by choosing the right set of codes. Just like today, you had to get the patient to sign an acknowledgment that he/she would be responsible for the costs of the cosmetic procedure.

My other patients told me this doctor could do this procedure in ten minutes.

As it turned out, I guess $75 for a procedure that took him about 10 minutes was not remunerative enough for him.

The procedure was performed. A month or two later she received a bill for $350 from the doctor's office.

She asked me about it and I said it had to be a mistake because I had learned the allowed amount for that type of minor procedure was around $75. I asked her to call the surgeon's office to see if they had charged her incorrectly or forgot to write off the unallowed part of the charge. The office was adamant and insisted that $350 was the amount she owed.

She was very worked up about this and I could not blame her because she existed on a very slender retirement income. So I called the surgeon and spoke to him personally. I reminded him this was not a cosmetic procedure. I suggested it could be rebilled under the diagnosis of infected cyst. I reminded him I'd sent her over because she was a diabetic and the lesion was tender, pink, and infected.

He said, "Bob, There's nothing I can do; I can't put the cyst back in."

For the rest of my career, I never sent this doctor another patient. I learned later that his office had had her sign a piece of paper that said she would pay the bill if the service were cosmetic. She had no idea what she had signed. She just trusted the doctor.

To be fair, maybe this incident did not reveal his true character. Maybe I caught him on a bad day. I wrote this story many years after the fact and I could not give him a chance to read my version of the events and make a comment or a correction. That's because he's dead now.

This situation is not as awful as the case I read in the news years ago. An ER doctor who discovered that a young black patient could not pay for the suturing job he had just performed and in anger, he snipped each suture. That left the wound gaping wide open. That guy lost his license.

Someone heard my patient's story and said I should have reported him to the state medical board.

The problem is that all he did was make a sleazy comment to me. In our system that is not actionable. He got the patient to sign the paper even if she did not understand what she was signing.

Being driven by the love of money is not one of the things for which you can lose your license. It takes more than that.

Would the Love of Money be a Type of Impairment in a Physician?

Avarice is a type of impairment, in my opinion. For sure, there are money-driven doctors who provide good care. We also have known there are doctors addicted to mind-numbing drugs who also provide good care 95% of the time.

I know there are more than a few doctors in private practice especially, who are barely making it. I know that's hard to believe. With financial pressure, they will feel a bias to make decisions to ensure their financial survival.

Let's say you are a doctor with $500,000 per year in obligations (mortgage, tuition, spousal demands, children's needs, medical school loans, staff at the office, rent, malpractice insurance) and then the insurance companies cut your payments. The contract you signed with them says you cannot bill the difference. Now despite the same amount of work, you are now bringing in $40,000 less. Before that you were just breaking even. Where are you going to get that $40,000? You are under financial stress despite a high income.

One day a salesman comes to the office and says for $50,000, he'll sell you a machine that will bring in $100,000 in lab test revenue every year. In your heart you have a good wolf and a bad wolf. The good wolf says, "You don't really need that machine. You've practiced good medicine without it." The bad wolf says, "It's legal, no one will criticize me. Even though this machine would not be as accurate as the lab to which I send specimens now, it's good enough. My nurse will learn to run it. The insurance companies will pay the patients' bills anyway."

The two wolves are fighting. You are pulled towards making a decision based on financial considerations over what's best for your patients.

This hypothetical doctor did not go into medicine to be rich. But if he buys that machine, he resembles the doctors who did. Society does not distinguish ethical from unethical medical practice based on motives. It judges based on the nature of the act itself. You should not say you did a bad thing for a good reason.

As a patient, the main thing is: be very careful when asked to sign something that says you will be responsible for the payment if insurance doesn't cover it. ☼ You need to find out why insurance won't cover it.

Government in Medicine.

You are told over and over again that people who rely on government payments would rather receive money than do work: you are outraged. On the other side of the political spectrum, you are told over and over again that what happened to your ancestors 200 years ago is why you are disadvantaged today: you are outraged.

In my experience, it's not cut and dried. Yes, there have been a lot of people who took advantage of social programs and others who genuinely needed them. Yes, some Americans would be millionaires today if their ancestors were not screwed out of what they had. And some are poor today because they have frittered away their ample inheritances. Who can say?

My grandparents, my parents, and likewise my wife and I never worked on researching our family tree. I'm quite sure that if I knew more about my roots, I would find some European ancestor who had been cheated out of what they had by somebody hundreds of years ago. My ancestors didn't come over to the New World because life was rosy in Europe.

As far as government windfalls go, it's not just the poor who benefit. God knows most doctors are recipients of government largess big time. Our educations are supported by government money including Medicare, significantly.

I remember about 15 years ago. It was a quiet Sunday morning and I was in the locker room after a swim. A man in his 70s was the weekend janitor. He always worked very slowly and always stopped his work to sit down and talk. That morning he said: "Doc, I think the government should get the hell out of healthcare, don't you agree?"

I did not hesitate. "Yes," I said. "Government has no business in healthcare. If I were you, I'd go home and write to Medicare. Tell them that you want to drop out effective immediately. Tell them to remove you from Medicare because the government has no business being in healthcare."

At that, he just stood up and went back to work.

We are so good at seeing that splinter in our neighbor's eye but cannot see the beam in our own.

Pascal's Wager For Philosophers, Physicists, and Fans of South Park as Well as Ordinary People

Pascal's Wager (as described in Wikipedia) is an argument in philosophy presented by the seventeenth-century French philosopher, mathematician, and physicist, Blaise Pascal (1623–1662). Pascal submits that humans bet with their lives whether God exists.

Did you think whether to consent to a coronary artery stent or bypass was a tough decision? Pascal thought whether to believe in God was a difficult one.

Pascal argues that a logical person should choose to believe in God. If God does not actually exist, such a person will have only a small loss (having given up some pleasures, some luxuries, etc.). But if God exists, he stands to receive immense gains (going to Heaven) and escape never-ending losses (an eternity in Hell). The argument also assumes that God will be angry with you if you fail to believe in Him and heap upon Him gobs and gobs of praise.

Pascal's Wager was based on the idea of the Christian God, though similar arguments have occurred in other religious traditions. The original wager was set out in Pascal's Pensées ("Thoughts") published after his death.

The next paragraph is from Alan Hájek, Stanford Encyclopedia of Philosophy.

"Historically, Pascal's Wager was groundbreaking as it had charted new territory in probability theory, was one of the first attempts to make use of the concept of infinity, marked the first formal use of decision theory, and anticipated the future philosophies of pragmatism and voluntarism."

Reader: I am not pretending to be an expert in philosophy. I'm a family doctor and much more down-to-earth. I had heard of Pascal's Wager years ago.

One day it just got to me. I was watching TV while on the treadmill at home. I was playing back some recorded episodes of South Park which I thought would entertain me as I exercised.

In July 2000, South Park had a two-episode story starting with "Do the Handicapped Go to Hell" and concluding with "Probably." For those who care about the details, this was Season 4, Episodes 10 and 11.

In the storyline, the boys hear that everyone is a sinner and will go to hell, but you can go to heaven instead provided you "confess your sins, eat crackers, and drink some wine." They decide it's time to go to church, take confession, etc.

The boys are concerned for their friend, Kyle because he is Jewish and for another friend, Timmy, because he is "handicapped." Timmy has a developmental issue and he can only say his name over and over. "Timmy!" "Timmy!" "Timmy!" "Timmy!" He says that all day. If that's all Timmy can say, how can he confess and be saved?

Kyle eventually is convinced that Jewish or not, he needs to go to church too. He goes home and talks to his parents.

Kyle: The guys said if I don't confess my sins and eat crackers, I'm gonna go to hell.

Sheila (Kyle's mother): Oh noooo, that's just Catholics. Us Jews don't believe in hell.

Kyle: We don't? But what if we're wrong?

Sheila: Well..., Kyle..., they could be wrong, too.

Kyle: Yeah, but if they're wrong, no big deal. If we're wrong, we burn in hell.

Gerald (Kyle's father): Kyle, it's all about being a good person now! You see, Christians use hell as a way to scare people into believing what they believe. **But to believe in something just because you're afraid of the**

consequences if you don't believe in something is no reason to believe in something. Understand?

Kyle: Well, you guys can do what you want! I'm going down to that church to confess my sins and eat crackers!

South Park does an excellent job explaining Pascal's Wager. It's risky to not believe in God. Kyle's father, Gerald refutes its logic with the marvelous line that sounds like doubletalk but isn't: "But to believe in something just because you're afraid of the consequences if you don't believe in something is no reason to believe in something." I'd like a T-shirt with that on it.

The object of the satire is obvious here. The authors mock those faiths that rely on fear of hell and damnation to motivate the behavior of their members. Good deeds should be motivated by either a divinely inspired desire to do good or a rational line of reasoning that directs us to do the same.

The medical profession often runs into decisions that resemble Pascal's Wager. Like certain religions, we doctors sometimes rely on fear of death to motivate our patients to accept our recommendations.

I don't think it wrong to point out to patients that death could be a consequence of a poor medical decision. But we're often too vague with these predictions of mortality.

I understand why doctors speak in vague terms. I remember learning about a doctor who proclaimed to his patient: "If you don't quit smoking, you'll be dead in five years." The patient left that doctor's practice, but five years later came by, wheeling his portable oxygen tank, just to say, "Tell the doctor, I'm still alive."

I don't think we should scare people with the prospect of death unless we can give them probability numbers so they can decide if the risk is reasonably significant, or significant enough to make a change. Like: "In five years if you quit smoking now your risk of dying would be halved."

Researchers have a lot of data they could use to generate such numbers, were there a demand for them by enough doctors seeking to motivate with facts rather than fear.

Why Are There Only Two Alternatives?

The more I think about it, I don't get what's so profound about Pascal's argument.

I think a lot of people understand this hell or no hell argument without knowing it's called "Pascal's Wager." Do we really need to adorn it with a fancy name? Maybe Pascal was the first to put this idea into words, so I suppose I should give him credit for that.

This writing must have been condemned by the Catholic Church as heretical in the 1600s. No wonder it was published only after Pascal had died.

What I don't understand is: Who said there are only two alternatives?

Pascal says either God doesn't exist or He does exist, and everything depends on those two polar opposites. In the first case, it doesn't matter if you don't believe. Or, in the second case, God exists and will eternally punish His creation, man, for not believing in Him, not engaging in certain rituals, and not praising Him.

What if there were a third possibility, or a fourth? What if God exists, takes an active role in judging and rewarding man, and has reserved hell only for those who violated one or more of the "Seven Deadly Sins."

How hell-worthy are these classic sins?

1. Sloth, which is laziness. I think that's not so deadly, although if enough people were too lazy to work, society would fall apart.

2. Gluttony, which means excessive eating. That's also bad for society; why should one person get fat while others starve? Should that warrant a ticket to hell?

3. Lust, which is a strong sexual desire. However, you really cannot control an emotional response. In theory, you can control how you behave, as opposed to what lustful thoughts might pop into your head. Maybe acting on lust, rather than experiencing the lustful desire, could be the criterion for being eternally punished.

4. Greed, which is an intense and selfish desire for something like wealth or power. Now that's something I think God would treat as a special punishment-worthy crime!

5. Envy, which is an unhappy longing for someone else's possessions, quality, or luck. I'm not sure that's bad enough to deserve being sent to hell. I say, "Quit wasting time, if you want something, work for it."

6. Wrath, which is anger. This is a big problem in God's world. It's such a negative emotion, and it often leads to hateful violence. Certainly, wrath would be a good reason for being hellbound.

7. Pride, which is defined as a feeling of deep pleasure or satisfaction derived from one's own achievements. That's kind of punishment-worthy because all your so-called accomplishments derive from God's gifts to you, don't they? I think you should be allowed to have a little pride. Just don't go overboard.

Benjamin Franklin aimed for twelve virtues for himself: Temperance, Silence, Order, Resolution, Frugality, Industry, Sincerity, Justice, Moderation, Cleanliness, Tranquility, and Chastity. I heard he was asked if he should have added "Humility." Franklin said that if he tried to be humble and succeeded, he'd just be proud that he had achieved another goal.

I would propose hypocrisy should be on the list of deadly sins. It would work like this: a person who says he believes in God but doesn't act like a good person would go to hell. People who do good deeds would be rewarded with eternal life. It wouldn't matter if they were of any religion or of no religion. It wouldn't matter if they know God, or praise God, or worship God, or even think about God.

Clearly, the lack of such other options affects the decision-making in the context of Pascal's Wager. The presumption that God punishes non-believers is a projection of a human-style personality onto God. This is a vision of a God with human emotions. Are His feelings actually hurt if He is not praised? We're talking about the God who created all those billions of galaxies astronomers see with space telescopes. Does He have time to worry about ingratitude let alone spend time being angry?

If God is God, then we cannot understand how He thinks. For all we know, God may only admit to heaven people who wear white socks with sandals. If that's the case, I'm in!!!

Likewise, in medical decision-making, the doctor may present only two alternatives from which to choose. Like Pascal did. So, ask about the other options.

And just in case hell is reserved for hypocrites and liars, let us in the medical profession refrain from pretending all our advice is based on proven science when so much of it is really based on hypotheses or educated guesses.

Those Monkeys Were In the Trees, Again

For older patients who are developing dementia, the future is bleak. Caregiver frustration and burnout are inevitable. The goal should be to delay caregiver burnout. There is no escaping that the patient will fail over time, but how long can we help keep the caregiver going?

One technique for delaying burnout is to abandon the idea of reasoning with the patient once reasoning stops working. Eventually, caregivers learn to stop arguing. I think in many cases attempting to reason with the patient could be abandoned a lot earlier.

A 55-year-old woman told the story about her 80-year-old mother who was having delusions or hallucinations due to dementia.

The daughter described how she hated going to visit her mother because they always argued about everything. The area of greatest disagreement was the mother's belief that there were monkeys outside her window playing in the trees.

They lived in Ohio. The daughter explained that monkeys live in warmer climates. She showed her mother proof by Googling nature references and maps that showed where monkeys lived in the world. She pointed out to her mother that nobody else could see these monkeys. To the same extent the daughter was persistent, the mother stubbornly maintained the monkeys were real. It was exhausting and frustrating for both of them. It was especially disappointing to the daughter because her mother had been such an intelligent and sensible person until this time in her life.

One day an idea came to the daughter. When her mother said, "I saw those monkeys outside yesterday playing in the trees."

The daughter simply said, "Wow! It's really early to see monkeys for this time of the year!"

The mother went on to the next topic; a conflict was avoided.

The daughter realized that the unhappy tragedy of her mother's dementia could not be fixed by arguing.

Here's another story, an unusual one, I would think. A ninety-three-year-old man was homebound and an aide came every day to help. She was about 40 years old, very kind, and dedicated. One of the required tasks was shower

ing. The old man had been stubborn all his life and now he was forgetful and lacked judgment. The patient would confuse his grandchildren with his children. He continued to be stubborn.

One day the aide said, "Time for your shower." The old man responded, "I'm not taking a shower today." The aide countered, "Well, if you're not taking a shower, then I guess I will. Wanna watch?" The patient popped right out of his chair and went to the bathroom. When he got there he had forgotten his objection to showering that day and he took his shower. The aide did not.

Is this a recommended approach? I doubt the nursing agency put that method in the manual. But it worked. It was creative.

Is there a comprehensive collection of approaches that solve the problem of caring for someone with Alzheimer's disease? No, not at all. These are just small tactics in a big battle.

The functional decline brought on by aging goes beyond Alzheimer's disease. Most of what older adults sometimes suffer memory-wise is just senescence, a normal but unfortunate change of aging.

It is the tradition in nearly all cultures and religions to help our parents as they age. In some places, it is a legal requirement to do so. But in the United States, the increase in two wage-earner families has made it more difficult to honor our ageing parents by helping in person.

The parents stay in their hometown; the kids move away. That used to be the exception. No longer. In many towns, more than half of those attending their 25th high school reunion come from out of town. Young people will go where the jobs are. And if we haven't moved away from our parents, sometimes our parents will have moved away from us.

Even if their children do live in town, a lot of parents don't want help. That doesn't mean they don't need it.

The Old Grandfather and His Grandson

This brief story is taken from the Grimm Brothers Tales (1812).

I have met more than one worker in the field of Geriatrics who had never heard this story. When I tell it to them, many of these specialists light up and say something like "I could use that." The point of the story is not subtle. I am retelling the story mostly in my own words.

There was once a very old man whose eyes had become dim, his ears were dull of hearing, and his knees trembled. He lived with his son and his son's wife and a four-year-old grandson. When the old man sat at the dinner table, he could hardly hold the spoon, and he would spill his soup upon the tablecloth or let it run out of his mouth.

His son and his son's wife were disgusted at this, so at last, the old grandfather was made to take his meals in the corner of the kitchen near the stove, and they gave him his food in an earthenware bowl. And he would look towards the table where the rest of the family ate with his eyes full of tears.

Once, too, his trembling hands could not hold the bowl, and it fell to the ground and broke. The young wife scolded him, but his son said nothing and only sighed. After that, they bought him a wooden bowl for a few half-pence, and he had to eat from the wooden bowl.

One day, the little grandson began to gather together some bits of wood he found outside. 'What are you doing there?' asked the father. 'I am making a little trough,' answered the child, 'for you and mother to eat from when I grow big.'

The man and his wife looked at each other for a while and began to cry. After that, they brought the old grandfather to the table, and from that day on, always let him eat with them, and likewise, they said nothing if he did spill anything or if something drooled from his mouth.

Being a Terran

What is a Terran? That's SiFi lingo for someone hailing from the planet Earth, as opposed to Mars or Venus. Citizens of those planets would be called Martians or Venusians.

I recall <u>I Love You to Death,</u> a 1990 film with Kevin Kline, Tracey Ullman, Joan Plowright, River Phoenix, William Hurt, and Keanu Reeves. In this comedy, each character is dumber than the next. In one scene Victoria Jackson asks Kevin Kline, who plays a philandering pizzeria owner if his Yugoslavian wife is Eurasian. "No," he says, "She's nota froma there."

It's hard to know what to call yourself in our melting pot society.

Genetically we are all mixed up which is a good thing.

For many people, I think it is bogus to identify with one particular country of origin. But it's always safe to call yourself a Terran. When you do, you are acknowledging that people are the same in the most important ways.

When you are a Terran, you can celebrate everybody's ethnic food as your own. People of all nations are your compadres. You can feel excitement in anticipation of all national holidays no matter what country is your origin. Hey! It's Bastille Day! (France). It's Guy Fawkes Day! (Britain). It's the Day of Reconciliation! (South Africa). And every two years, whoever wins the Olympic event you are watching, will surely be one of your people. Terrans have won every Olympic Gold Medal since the first modern Olympics in 1896.

So I prefer to think of myself as a Terran, ethnically. And did I mention we have our own special holiday: Earth Day?

Being a Descendent of Eve

How can it be that we are all the same and yet all different? Every person on earth other than identical twins has their own unique nuclear DNA. That's the DNA in the chromosomes within the nucleus. Nuclear DNA is what makes you who you are, genetically. It's unique because it comes from the combining of the DNA from the mother's egg and the father's sperm. Even people with the same parents have unique DNA combinations, except for identical twins. Every sibling born to that couple results from a unique mixture of the parents' DNA.

But there is also DNA in the mitochondria of each cell. Mitochondria are the energy centers of our cells. We don't get mitochondria from our fathers. The mitochondria come from our mother's egg. Every time a cell divides into two, each half gets some of the many mitochondria, which in turn divide within the cell to prepare for the cell's next division. Your mitochondrial DNA comes directly and only from your mother. She got it from her mother, who got it from her mother, and so on and so on. Scientists believe all human mitochondrial DNA traces back to one woman, who could be called "Mitochondrial Eve."

It does not matter from where your ancestors came. English, Chinese, Indian, American, or African, etc., we all have pretty much the same mitochondrial DNA.

So it follows there was a single original female human being from which we all descended. She gave all humans alive today the mitochondrial DNA we now all possess in common. In the Bible, the original mother is called Eve. Genesis could be very close to being accurate, with just a small problem: Adam. In order to have possessed human mitochondrial DNA, Adam would had to be Eve's son. Just a small detail. Luckily God doesn't have to obey the laws of science,

Back to being a Terran. We are all different but we are all the same in the sense that we all have nearly the same Mitochondrial DNA. On the other hand, we are all uniquely mixed up as far as our Nuclear DNA goes.

Often patients disclose their ethnic background. The self-stated racial classification of the patient is frequently wrong. They advertise this fact on TV when they push genetic testing kits. I love the one where the man says, "We thought we were Swedish but we went to Sweden and found out we are Norwegian!."

Rather than the genetics of the patient, it's important for doctors to know something about the cultural background of the patient. Culture trumps genetics.

Monkeys and Welshmen

Years ago I had a patient who was from Romania. He spoke with an accent. He was a brilliant man, a Ph.D., a university professor in a scientific field. He was also stern. I had patients who had been taught by him. He was respected by his students, but also feared. I never knew him to make small talk or to kid around.

But one day when I walked into the exam room, he suddenly opened our visit by asking me 'whether I knew that most people came from monkeys, but not Welshmen.' I was curious about this non-Darwinian way of thinking.

Naturally, I said: "Where do Welshmen come from?"

He said, "Wales."

Since then, everybody who tells me they are part Welsh gets to hear this story.

Understanding Culture Beats Understanding Genetics

I've been privileged to care for people from many different lands. I remember one gentleman who was from a country in Africa. He was of the Muslim faith. He told me there was really no point in working on his diabetes because what was going to happen "had already been written." He could not alter the fate that diabetes had handed him. So he did not work on his diet or take his medicine regularly. Nevertheless, he came for the pills.

That philosophy made it pretty difficult to get him to change his diet. Following the right diet is the most difficult intervention in patients with Type 2 diabetes.

By the way, one thing I love about Muslims is that mostly there is no drinking alcohol. That makes life ever so much easier for a doctor; it's too bad some Muslims drink despite the Qur'an categorizing it as unlawful.

Believing the future is fixed by God is called "preordination" This idea that all future events are preordained by God is believed by parts of Christianity, Judaism, and Islam.

I was unwilling to believe this might be rigidly written into the Muslim faith. A few days later I saw another Muslim patient and I asked him his opinion on whether his religion specifies that the future is already written.

Before I tell you how the second Muslim patient answered my question I want to discuss some scenes from a movie. I remember one poignant part of the classic film Lawrence of Arabia. Lawrence is out trying to cross the huge Sinai desert with his army of Arab freedom fighters. Lawrence's new friend Gassim has fallen behind the group and is lost in the desert. Lawrence rides back, risking his life to save his friend after rejecting the advice that Gassim's death "Was already written."

Lawrence ignores that fatalistic prediction and launches into the impossibly empty desert. Defying the odds, he finds Gassim and brings him back to safety. Lawrence did not accept the concept of "It is written."

A few scenes later, however, Gassim has been in a fight and murdered a man from a different tribe. This dispute has divided the expeditionary force. To save his army from breaking apart in tribal strife, it is necessary for Lawrence as commander, to execute Gassim in front of the whole company. "It was written," that Gassim would die after all.

So is it written?

A Muslim friend told me that even if something were written, through prayer, God could change it. I guess some things are may be written, but maybe it is also written that God expects us to try to make things better on this planet.

With this recollection, I asked the second Muslim patient, whether there is any use in taking care of your health if your fate is "written." What does the Qur'an say about that?

He told me the Qur'an says our bodies are a gift from Allah and to respect Him we must take care of that gift, we must protect our body, and our health.

I think this might be the quote from that holy text that applies. "Taking proper care of one's health is the right of the body."

So, I appreciate another part of Islam.

I think there are more things in common than there are important differences among these major religions.

A Good Physician Cannot Ignore Culture and Language

Some patients don't speak English. In central Ohio, we have many immigrants from Africa, from the Middle East, and from Nepal. For those that don't speak English, doctors' offices have interpreters. In medical interpreting, the interpreter sometimes has to clarify to make the meaning exact. A translator works on the written documents. Patients need interpreters who interpret not just the words that they said, but what they mean. There's a difference.

Idiomatic expressions are even harder to interpret than words. We hosted a German exchange student in 2000-1. Markus spoke pretty good English when he came to us. I realized he would need more help with idiomatic expressions than with ordinary words and phrases.

One day we were watching something on TV. My wife came into the room and asked Markus a question. He got up and moved a few feet to answer her. He stopped directly between my eyes and the television.

I said, "Markus, you make a better door than a window."

He looked at me with a puzzled look. Suddenly he smiled and said, "I know what you're saying, Bob. In German, we have a similar expression. We say 'It's obvious your father wasn't a glassmaker.'"

During the last five years of my career, I was working for Ohio State University at a Family Medicine office. We had the privilege of caring for many Nepali refugee patients, sometimes several on the same day. We were told our office cared for more Nepali patients than any of the other OSU branch offices.

With refugees, as with all patients, most new patients come to you because of word of mouth.

When I came to OSU in 2012 and met the first of these patients, I asked my colleagues, "How did these Nepali people get here?"

No one knew much. Everyone knew they were refugees and they were Hindus but not much more. Some of the people at the office said they were Bhutanese, not Nepali. Other than that, nobody knew their story.

For most of these patients, we needed interpreters. Each visit with a Nepali patient took at least twice as long. Asking "Does your throat hurt when you swallow?" could take 2 minutes to get an answer. There was no time for small talk like "How did it happen you came here as a refugee?"

As I mentioned, there is a difference between "translator" and "interpreter." In English, a translator means converting written text from one language to the next. An interpreter converts oral language.

But medical interpreters may have to do more than convert words. Sometimes they need to use different or additional words and phrases to get the meaning across.

After seeing a few Nepali patients and struggling to help them, I did some research. I learned their history and shared it with all the other doctors at the office.

Nepalese started settling in nearby Bhutan as early as 1620. In the 20th century, many more settled in southern Bhutan which had been fairly uninhabited. They farmed the land. Southern Bhutan became the most important food-producing area of the country. But these Nepalese were Hindu people and Bhutan was a Buddhist country. The Nepali Bhutanese never assimilated, nor did they become citizens.

The government of Bhutan became concerned about the large number of Nepalese living in their south. At the same time, the Nepalese began agitating for basic rights.

Between 1990 and 1993, after considerable political turmoil as well as physical strife including murders, assaults, rapes, and forced marches, over 100,000 Bhutanese people of Nepali origin were forced to walk to Nepal from Bhutan. Most had never been to their "home" country before.

Under the authority of the United Nations High Commissioner for Refugees, the families were settled in camps in Nepal.

You could see these camps via the internet. If you zoomed in on Google Earth you could find them. In the beginning, the camps' occupants were subject to overcrowding, epidemic diseases, and malnutrition. Over the first decade, the conditions improved. The younger people were schooled. I have read that the schooling offered in the camps was actually better than that offered Nepali citizens in the surrounding countryside.

But the older farmers had never been to school. The Bhutanese government had made it illegal for the Nepali language to be taught in schools.

Eventually, eight of the world's best countries took in these refugees: Australia, Canada, Denmark, New Zealand, the Netherlands, Norway, the United Kingdom, and the USA. By "best" I mean if countries were to be measured in kindness. Our nation has been privileged to take over seven times as many as the other seven combined(2015 stats).

The kids from these families spoke English pretty well because they grew up going to school in the refugee camps. But the older farmers uniformly did not learn English. They were the best farmers in Bhutan, but their language skills were at the bottom. They couldn't write or read in their own language. They had not needed skill in language. I don't think they had very extensive vocabularies in any subjects besides farming. They had no experience with doctors and had few medical words in their command to communicate with modern medical professionals.

The Nepali interpreters, themselves refugees now employed doing this work, struggled to get the concepts across. As their doctors, we struggled to understand the symptoms of our patients.

When I asked if the patient had "diarrhea" I heard the interpreter use the word "diarrhea." Several interpreters told me there was no word in their language to describe diarrhea.

Another problem was distinguishing pain from tenderness. In medicine when something hurts we call it pain but when it hurts to touch it, we call that tenderness. Almost no Nepali patients could not distinguish pain from tenderness when giving a history.

Me: Is your elbow tender?

(Interpreter spending a minute conversing in Nepalese.) Yes, doctor, the elbow has been hurting for two weeks.

Me: But is it painful only when you touch it or does it hurt all the time?

(Interpreter conversing with the patient another minute.)

Yes doctor the elbow is painful for two weeks now.

I concluded after talking with the interpreters that they just did not have the word for tenderness, so they did not appreciate the concept of tenderness. It was just hurt.

I never had to do so much guessing in my entire career. I would bring patients back again and again if nature hadn't healed them. In one case the patient had something hurting in the mid-abdomen. Was the discomfort there all the time or intermittently? Not clear. Was it sharp or dull or burning? Not clear. What made it worse or better? Not clear. Many other questions were asked. Nothing was clear.

Let's try something that lowers the acid in the stomach and come back in ten days. Ten days later, no better. Let's try something else. Finally, after three visits I ordered tests. What should I order? A gallbladder study? Too specific. That's just the gallbladder. An endoscopy? Too specific. That's just the esophagus, stomach, and duodenum. What did I do? I ordered blood tests and a CT of the chest and abdomen.

The insurance company required a preauthorization for the CT scan. I had to talk to a nurse and then a doctor.

Insurance Rep: Why do you want to do a CT scan?

Me: Because after three visits I know something is wrong but I can't get a decent history.

Insurance Rep: That's not listed in our guidebook as an acceptable reason to justify the CT study.

Me: I know, but I'm stuck. I know something is wrong. I explained the language barrier.

Then unexpectedly... the insurance company's doctor approved the CT scan.

The scan was done. Unfortunately, the scan revealed the patient had an advanced cancer. It had been going on for many months. He died not long after that.

It wasn't just language that delayed the diagnosis. He grew up in a culture in which early symptoms were endured rather than reported. Had he spoken English or had a cultural background that would have led him to seek medical care earlier... who knows if the outcome would have been different?

To Be Understood By Your Physician You May Need to Share Your Social Background and Your Personal Story.

It was easy to divide the Nepali patients into two groups: There were the younger people who spoke English, worked, and were having children and starting the American dream. Most were becoming citizens and a few had purchased homes. The other group was the older patients, the ones whose visits took twice as long to accomplish half as much due to the language problem. They often dressed in colorful, traditional garb, as you would see in pictures of people in India. They would always start the visit by smiling and saying "Namaste." When I asked about what they had done in Bhutan they would all say "farmer."

They seemed to have lived similar lives. They had farmed. They had raised children. That life ended when they had been forced to walk hundreds of miles from Bhutan to Nepal, leaving behind farms and farm animals. They had lived in camps for two decades in rows of identical huts. Now they had finally come to America.

But I learned that to truly understand them you had to appreciate that they were not all cast from the same mold. Most seemed to be of a middle class of pleasant, bright people who had worked hard until their lives were upturned by forces they could not control.

But others were from an upper class. The women wore thicker gold chains with their traditional gowns. The men dressed with a touch of elegance too. Their medical histories included tests and treatments at medical centers in India where they had gone for specialist care. These patients were more assertive about their medical care.

I also recognized a small number who could be described as a lower class. They had more medical conditions related to abuse or neglect or self-abuse such as sexually

103

transmitted infections. Some were the wives of husbands who had gone overseas for work and never returned. They had not owned farms in Bhutan. They were not connected socially to the population that I thought was like a middle class.

My research into the history of these patients only reached a superficial depth, I know. But I think what I learned helped me understand how to better serve as their doctor. The experience of caring for Nepali immigrants amplified for me the importance of understanding the patients' skills in language, patterns defined by social class, and cultural norms.

I had an American-born patient once who shared with me that he had been convicted of manslaughter and had served time in prison. Now he was running his own business. After learning that from him, I always considered him a person I could admire for getting his life on track, and I rooted for his success.

Don't hesitate to share with your personal physicians your social background, your education, and your personal story. ☼

I Wasn't Very Familiar With My Own Culture

Don't assume your doctor is aware of everyday things outside of the realm of medicine. Sometimes we doctors don't know our own world.

It's unbelievable how clueless a doctor can become in a quarter of a century while he or she is busy in training and then in practice and also raising children. That was true in my case. When I took the Medical College Achievement Test, which you needed to apply to medical school, I scored at the 99th percentile for the category of general knowledge. That means I scored more points than 99 of 100 premedical students taking the test. I think that was because I had a wide range of interests and always read more than what school required. But I have a dismal level of knowledge of popular culture between 1968 and 1999. I was too busy in college, medical school, residency, and then starting practices and raising small children for pop culture.

Trivia games with references to a TV show from the late '60s and '70s? Don't ask me. I never saw Star Trek until it was on reruns. Ditto for MASH. We did have a TV in our dorm at Princeton. It didn't work. It was just an accessory for the room. We thought it looked good. We also had a freezer inside of our fridge that had so much frost build-up that only one soda pop can could fit.

Years after Star Trek was on TV, I was surprised to learn that Captain Kirk has three ears. Not Spock with the pointy ears, I mean Kirk. I didn't know that. He has his left ear, he has his right ear, and he has "Space" the final front ear. They tell you that at the beginning of every show.

In 1992 there was to be a medical conference in Cincinnati that coincided with the 25th anniversary of my graduation from high school in a Cincinnati suburb. This reunion was to be a showcase of my cluelessness.

I remember our class had had a 15th reunion which I didn't attend. Someone had sent me the program afterward. I felt bad because I never told anyone in the class my current address and I was listed as "care of" my mother since they had her address. A lot of people already knew that address well because we lived across the street from the high school. I thought my classmates probably saw that "care of mother" address and thought I was dwelling in my mother's basement or maybe my mail just went there because I was an inmate in some institution.

In retrospect, I was an inmate in the institution of medicine.

My mother had moved to California in 1985, so it was unlikely that I would receive a forwarded invitation to the 25th reunion. I didn't even know whether we were going to have a 25th reunion. But one day in November 1991 it popped into my head we were due for the 25th that summer and I wrote the school. Several months later I got an invitation to come to the class reunion. And when I found out there was a conference the same weekend in the same city I signed up for both. Busy doctors with children look for these dual-purpose trips.

When I signed in at the reunion that evening, my classmate at the table said, "Bob, it's because of YOU we are having this reunion! You wrote a letter to the school and the Principal's office made inquiries. No one had thought about this reunion until you wrote that letter. So we're here because of you!"

In high school, I had been was pretty busy with class work and my sport, swimming, and in retrospect, I was pretty shy and didn't really make close friends there. It didn't help that I had only joined the class at the end of my sophomore year. I had stayed in New Jersey six weeks after my family left for Ohio because my swim team was headed

106

for a state swimming title. I only had a few weeks of my sophomore year in Ohio.

The first summer after coming to Cincinnati, I had creamed a city swimming record and maybe it was for that reason that a lot of people knew my name by my junior year. It's bad to be a shy 16-year-old where everybody knows your name. I mean, usually, you don't have a clue what their name is. What do you say when they say, "Hello, Bob." Maybe: "Oh hello, you there."

Part of the reason I was shy in those years was because my father was dying from cancer and his treatments had started at that time. I dreaded talking about that with anyone my age. You know...boys don't cry.

But I volunteered as the student photographer for the yearbook and the school newspaper. I had photographed a lot of my classmates. I had seen their faces come up in the developing trays in my darkroom. They had seen the camera covering my face.

Anyway, here I was at the reunion, walking about and talking to classmates I had not known that well 25 years earlier.

I saw a fellow named Jim. We had had several classes together including honors English and honors math. I don't think they called it honors this or that in those days; it was just the class into which all the academically top kids were placed. They gave us more work.

The main thing I remembered about Jim was that he had gone to Harvard. I sat down next to him and said something like, "Hi Jim, how's it going? What did you do after graduating from Harvard?"

Becoming a family doctor had taught me the art of conversation. I would never have been able to put together such an eloquent pair of conversation openers when I was in high school. But in medical school they taught me the technique of talking to people.

Jim told me that he had opened a microbrewery.

I said something like, "Wow, that sounds like a lot of fun; what did you do after that?

I had just assumed that such an exciting adventure into the world of beer-making would have been short-lived.

And then he said something like, "Well we expanded and I purchased a lot more capacity and I guess you could say what I do is I brew and sell beer."

I said, "Wow! Great! Tell me the name of your beer. Maybe I've heard of it."

He told me the name but I hadn't heard of it. I hadn't had much to do with beers or bars in my sheltered medical and family life. I confessed I had never heard of his beer. I told him that if I ever did see it, I would think of him.

Then I went on to talk to another classmate.

Later I recognized the name of Jim's beer when I read about him in the Wall Street Journal. His beer is called Sam Adams. As of 2021, Jim Koch's company is the 9th largest brewery in the United States. He's the guy in the TV commercials who talks about the hops. He's the brewer, the pioneer of craft brewing. He's the guy whose beer I had never known in 1992. Talk about clueless!

We Have Our Own Witch Doctors: Supplements

"The witch doctor succeeds for the same reason all the rest of us succeed. Each patient carries his own doctor inside him. We are at our best when we give the doctor who resides within each patient a chance to go to work." Albert Schweitzer.

Dr. Albert Schweitzer, who's that? If you are in the younger part of the population you may never have heard of him. He was like the Mother Teresa of the 1950s. He won the Nobel Peace Prize in 1952. He was a musicologist and organist who became a theologian who next became a doctor at age 37 and went to Africa to found a hospital in Gabon. That's where he spent the rest of his life.

I read this story about him from Do You Believe In Magic by Paul Offit MD. This is a most interesting book about alternative medicine which I highly recommend. Offit took his story from The Anatomy of an Illness as Perceived by the Patient by Norman Cousins.

Norman Cousins was an author, editor, advocate for world peace, and a man who cured his own autoimmune disorder with laughter and then went on to lecture about using laughter as a treatment in medicine.

Mr. Cousins went to visit Dr. Albert Schweitzer in Africa. According to the story, Cousins was a guest at Dr. Schweitzer's hospital and said something to the effect, "Without you, the people here would have to rely on the witch doctor."

Dr. Schweitzer asked something like, "How much do you know about witch doctors? Tomorrow we'll pay ours a visit."

The next day they left the hospital and went through the jungle to a clearing where the local witch doctor saw patients. With his permission, they watched the witch doctor work for two hours.

Dr. Schweitzer explained that the witch doctor took care of a lot of patients who had conditions that tended to go away on their own. He treated them with herbs to make into teas. A second type of patient he treated with "African psychotherapy." The third type of patient had more "substantial" problems that would benefit from "modern medicine." Those patients were sent to Dr. Schweitzer's hospital.

Most herbal "supplements" are unproven in the treatment of disease. They are the European/ American equivalent of the witch doctor.

Sorry to those I offend. Most of what you read about what these supplements do for you is made up. With vitamins, just because a deficiency disease can be cured by a supplement, it does not mean that the benefits keep increasing when you increase the dose higher and higher. It's like a life preserver when the boat has sunk. One life preserver keeps you at the level of the water. Two or three or four life preservers and you're still at the water level. Those extra life preservers don't allow you to float 10 feet above the water. It's the same thing with extra vitamins.

The fact that I am knocking supplements does not mean I am some kind of tool of the pharmaceutical industry. I'm not. I'm no fan. Too many products of Big Pharma are barely effective, have unacceptable side effects, are not better than what's already available, and are over-promoted and over priced.

Patients want modern medicine for everything but there are plenty of conditions that do not require it. Many patients won't accept the advice to wait.

Doctor: "Let's see if your body will cure you."

The patient looks dismayed.

So the doctor gives placebos.

Not the classic placebo, which is a sugar pill disguised to look like the real thing.

Rather, we give a largely ineffective drug that won't harm the patient while waiting for nature to do the job.

Voltaire: Entertain the patient while nature heals him.

Doctors: If it's the only thing that will help them, let's choose placebos that are both inexpensive and harmless for these patients.

Let's also remember the placebo can be very powerful. As Schweitzer said, "We are at our best when we give the doctor who resides within each patient a chance to go to work."

Carmen Married Mr. Cohen

There was a lady whose last name was Carmen who married a man named Cohen. Then she divorced him and then took back her maiden name, Carmen. Then she married his brother and once again she was Mrs. Cohen. Next she divorced him and took back the name Carmen. After a while, her friends didn't know whether she was Carmen or Cohen.

A nice doctor from the Middle East saw my joke online and commented:

She wrote, "Well, a Cohen (a name retained for the high clergy who were at the Temple in Jerusalem) is not allowed to marry a divorcee (in a Jewish wedding, at least, not a secular procedure), so actually the brother couldn't have married her..."

Me: "That's good to know, but if I made the first brother die so that the other brother could marry the widow, that would have been a bit sad for a joke. Thanks for the informative comment."

Nice Doctor: "Yeah, kill the bastard! There's no prohibition over a widow."

Me: "Yes, I guess it would be nicer if the first Cohen would die of natural causes for the sake of the joke."

I never knew that Cohen was a surname that implied so many rules.

When I think of this joke I recall my doctor when I was a kid.

"Rub Vicks On His Chest"

My pediatrician was named Dr. Cohen.

It was 1960. I was about 10 and I had a bad chest cold. My mother took me in. Dr. Cohen determined I had bronchitis, which is nearly always a virus. He advised my mother to rub Vicks VapoRub (mentholated petrolatum) on my chest.

I had been reading this and that about science and had just learned something about DMSO (Dimethyl sulfoxide) which penetrates the skin so deeply that it enters the bloodstream. After rubbing it on your skin you can taste it in a few minutes.

I asked Dr. Cohen something like, "How could the Vicks get into my lungs." I said that if it passed through the skin, "it would go through blood vessels on the way to my lungs and some of it would go around in the bloodstream until it reached my taste buds and then I'd taste it." But I stated that clearly, when people put Vicks on the skin, they do not taste menthol. So the Vicks on the chest wouldn't get into the lungs, I reasoned. That was the gist of what I told him.

I expressed these doubts to my doctor as respectfully as a respectful ten-year-old could.

Dr. Cohen didn't bat an eye. I recall his exact words. He said, "That's not how it works. It just gives your mother something to do while Nature heals you."

I never forgot what he said. It was disarmingly honest and represented something that medicine so often lacks. Later I figured out that he understood the power of the body to heal itself. He chose the option of putting away the prescription pad for a case of viral bronchitis. He was not only a doctor, he was a teacher.

But many users of Vicks for a chest cold will believe it works because you get better.

Cause and Effect, in that Order

Ambrose Bierce in the Devil's Dictionary defined "EFFECT, n. The second of two phenomena which always occur together in the same order. The first, called a Cause, is said to generate the other—which is no more sensible than it would be for one who has never seen a dog except in the pursuit of a rabbit to declare the rabbit the cause of a dog."

A chest massage with Vicks might soothe the suffering patient psychologically, and in theory that could help the immune system. But can one say it was the massage or just the attention paid to the patient that helped? Maybe you could have used Crisco instead of Vicks

In other words, you might get better after a series of Vicks chest massages but that would not prove the Vicks and the relief of cold symptoms had a cause and effect relationship.

I never forgot what Dr. Cohen taught me at age ten. But 13 years later in medical school, it occurred to me that healing may be affected by the act of soothing or reassuring or simply paying attention to the suffering of the patient. So low-tech treatments may work, not because of a pharmacologic effect, but from a psycho-physiological reaction. I'll restate that in plain language. Low-tech treatments may work like a placebo or like the witch doctor. They don't directly improve your body chemistry. They work by affecting your mind. The mighty mind fixes the body.

We get into trouble when we apply the higher-risk hi-tech diagnostics and therapeutics to problems that will resolve on their own. Let's remember how Dr. Schweitzer used his Witch Doctor.

Don't immediately jump for the high tech stuff when the problem may go away on its own or with benign treatments.

The old doctors taught me time will heal. They called this "tincture of time."

Learning From Our Mistakes

Oscar Wilde wrote, "Experience is the name everyone gives to their mistakes."

He was only partly right in my opinion. You can't claim to be "experienced" unless you have *learned something* from your mistakes.

In employment want ads we see, "Experience required." We don't see, "Candidates must have made a lot of mistakes."

The ads could have said, "Candidates must have made a lot of mistakes or studied the mistakes of others and have learned how to avoid error." But that's too many words.

I bring up this topic because in medicine we should learn from our bad outcomes. That can be difficult because the public prefers to believe we don't make mistakes.

Doctors and nurses like to believe it too. So do our employers.

One kind of error arises from a lack of information. I believe the people who write patient education materials don't often enough relate stories of patients who did poorly because they lacked information. They give information for sure. How often do they make their information interesting by presenting stories about what can happen to patients who did not know what they needed to know.

Let's consider the standard advice on the prevention of influenza.

You hear this on the radio and on television and you see it on billboards and on TV public service announcements. "Get your flu shot." "Cover your cough." "Wash your hands." Less often do they say "Do not touch your eyes or nose."

During the Covid-19 pandemic did you ever hear anyone say, "Your mask can help you because it stops you from touching your nose where the virus enters the body." I did not.

Did you see on TV anything like this? "This patient is dying. He has been in the intensive care unit for a week with Covid. It started when he rubbed his eyes."

You can't get into a building by walking through the walls. You have to use the doors. The respiratory viruses get into the body thru your nose or your eyes. That's the only doorway that works for them. Respiratory viruses only come in through the eyes or nose.☼

Not touching the face should be the number one thing you are taught. ☼

How did it happen that washing your hands is ranked above "Don't touch your nose or eyes?" It's curious.

I hope that Covid is past us by the time you read this. So let's discuss influenza which has the same mode of transmission.

Influenza enters the body through an eye or the nose. It does not infect us by entering through the skin of the hands. Unless you just washed those hands immediately before touching your nose or your eyes, you may catch influenza regardless of how many other times per day you washed your hands. You could wash every five minutes until your hands crack and bleed from repeated exposure to the soap and water or hand cleaner.

But if you get a good bit of flu virus on those "just washed" hands and then touch your eyes or nose, you can get influenza. If you're not a face toucher, you can have influenza virus on your hands at 9 a.m. and not wash until noon and you won't infect yourself, as long as you are careful to keep your hands away from your nose and eyes and don't let people cough or sneeze on you.

To put it backwards, here is HOW TO CATCH influenza.

Step 1: Wash your hands, dry them,

Step 2: Before the next time you wash, touch something an infected person touched to get some virus on your hand;

Step 3: Rub your eyes or rub your nose. Rubbing is just one option: also scratch, pick, touch, etc.

Step 4: Wash your hands again. Feel good about washing your hands like they tell you on TV.

The deed is done. You have inoculated yourself with influenza. Now whether or not you get sick depends on the size of the inoculation, and the strength of your immune system. Maybe your immune system has some B lymphocytes that remember your flu shot three years ago when a similar flu was the active strain in the vaccine. In that case, you might get lucky and only get a mild infection.

Washing your hands even one minute after inoculating your eye or nose would not have saved you. The barn door was closed but the horse had already left the barn.

The first message in these campaigns should be "Don't touch your face." The second message should be when you see that someone's about to sneeze or cough quickly turn your head in the opposite direction. The stream of influenza-containing droplets from the sick person will crash innocently into the back of your head. Influenza germs on the back of your head have missed the portal of entry.

It's gross to think about someone's droplets landing on the back of your head but it's better than on your face.

117

One could argue that handwashing is important because it can stop the spread of virus particles to many different surfaces. One could also argue that despite being coached many times not to touch your nose or eyes, people do it anyway.

I think the dominance of hand washing advice for influenza prevention is with us because hospital people have been writing up the patient education materials. Most hospital infections are spread by dirty hands. Droplets are of lesser concern for the hospital-acquired infections which these infection control people spend their lives trying to stop.

So the story we should teach: "George was sick with influenza for a week because he rubbed his eyes and his nose."

A Talking Parrot

Once there was a polite, insecure man who lived alone. He always wanted to have a parrot and teach it to talk but he was afraid to buy one. What if he couldn't teach it to speak? If it never learned to talk, he'd be stuck with it and parrots can live 100 years. Full of self-doubt, he never bought the parrot.

Years passed. One day he saw an ad for a parrot whose owner had already taught it to speak. He bought it sight unseen without learning anything about the background of the creature. The parrot was delivered. It could certainly talk, and it talked all day long, but every other utterance was a four-letter word.

It must have been raised in a sailors' bar, he concluded.

This very nice man couldn't tolerate the profanities. He tried everything to get the parrot to stop cursing. He played soft music. He scolded it when it cursed. If the parrot went five minutes without an obscenity, he rewarded it with a treat. But his efforts were to no avail. The cursing continued unabated.

The man was embarrassed to have people come to his home. He felt he was stuck.

One day he was so frustrated that he took the parrot out of the cage, threw it into the freezer and closed the door.

After a few minutes, he felt guilty. A parrot is a tropical animal. He knew it couldn't survive long in that cold.

So he opened the door of the freezer and the parrot hopped onto his arm, looked him straight in the eye, and said,

"Sir, I wish to apologize for my behavior. I promise you I will never say those bad words again."

The man was flabbergasted and didn't know how to respond, so he just said,

"OK, err..... good."

Then the parrot spoke again, "If I may be bold enough to enquire... what did the turkey do?"

An Object Lesson

The consequences of your action or inaction may be more serious than you anticipate. It is lucky if you get the type of shocking warning that we would call an object lesson.

Maybe you don't get thrown into a freezer. But you get "burned" from your mistake.

Sometimes you don't get a warning.

You could get burned the first time you made the mistake. You get that speeding ticket the first time you take your parents' car out by yourself.

You can learn from your mistakes but it's much better if you can learn from the mistakes of others instead.

Seek to educate yourself about bad things that can happen and then learn to steer clear of those situations.

A patient can learn from the errors of other patients. A doctor can learn from the errors of other doctors.

The Study of Error

When I was 37 I became Chair of the Department of Family Practice at our 500-bed community hospital. At the time, I was young for a department chair, in fact, I was the second youngest attending physician in the entire department.

This was a time when "Quality Improvement" and "Patient Safety" were concepts yet to be developed. We had committees dealing with this type of thing though. In 1987 we called it the "Patient Care Committee." Later it was the "Quality Assurance Committee" and a few years later I renamed it the "Quality Improvement Committee."

I was the first residency-trained Family Doctor at our hospital. I had been trained at one of the oldest Family Medicine residency programs in the U.S. I was in the fourth class of residents to enter that program.

Two years before I was appointed Chair, I was asked to be Vice-Chair, a job that entailed going to one meeting a month if the "Chief" was out of town.

The Chair of the department was Dr. Harold Chevlen. When he was a young doctor, Dr. Chevlen had delivered a baby.

The baby grew up, went to school, got a job at a hospital as a dietitian and I married her. Most doctors don't have the

120

chance to learn from someone who had once spanked their wife.

For the younger readers, gently spanking the bottom was what they did after a baby was born in those days. They thought it would encourage the baby to take its first breath.

I decided I should attend the monthly "Patient Care Committee." Dr. Chevlen said, "Go to those meetings. You'll learn something."

It was kind of a sad meeting. The data analyst would bring charts within which someone had found "problems." We did not call them errors or mistakes.

The chair of the committee, a senior family doctor (and a wonderful person I should mention) would look at the information in the chart and nearly always say, "Well he's a good doctor and he must have had a reason for doing/ not doing that, but he didn't put it in the progress notes as he should have, so let's sign off that chart as a documentation issue." I can still hear him reciting that most non-confrontational conclusion.

I recall about 1985 I cornered the hospital's CEO at a reception and told him I thought the big challenge of the next decade was going to be Quality of Care, not Finance. He looked at me as though I were some kind of unusual insect. He did not say a word.

Two years later I was named Chief. This was the start of a long segment of my career. I spent about 14 years as Chair of the Family Medicine Department and then the next seven years as a Vice President of Medical Affairs.

By this time, my prediction about quality was coming true.

In 1987 the big challenge was how to implement quality medical care. It was hard to define quality let alone determine how a doctor in leadership could improve quality.

My boss was Dr. Gene Butcher, the Vice President of Medical Affairs, a great internist in the opinion of many including myself. During our first meeting after I had been appointed Chair, he opened up the Joint Commission manual and read to me where it said that the Chair of the Department was responsible for the quality of the work done by the doctors in the department.

I said, "How in the hell am I supposed to do that?"

You should understand that our department was 95% composed of self-employed physicians. People don't listen to you as carefully when you are not the person who signs their paychecks.

Dr. Butcher said, "That's what you have to figure out."

I had to improve the quality of the work done by the department. People would say: "What is quality? The answer was, "Well, it's like what the Supreme Court said about pornography. You know it when you see it." That wasn't a good enough definition.

I finally decided that quality was not an absolute thing, it was a comparative.

It was like diamonds. You think your slightly imperfect diamond was a top-quality gem until you see a VVS or nearly flawless one at a better jewelry store.

Quality was the absence of flaws in diamonds. In medicine, we call those flaws by another name: "Errors."

In the late 80s during a hospital Joint Commission inspection at the hospital, I asked the inspectors how do we best study quality of care in Family Medicine? Their answer: "We don't have any good indicators for Family Medicine." An indicator would be a single facet of care on which you could compile statistics: like how many drug interactions were missed or how often a low potassium level was not treated.

The inspectors were of no help. But it was soon clear to me that quality was about reducing errors.

Studying on my own, I had read about the work of a professor at the Harvard School of Public Health, Dr. Lucien Leape. He had published a five-page report on the subject which I probably read fifty times. Dr. Leape was as eloquent as Shakespeare to me.

Around this time the Japanese were revolutionizing the way autos were manufactured. Workers were rewarded for finding mistakes. Anyone who found one was empowered to stop the production line. That way the flaw could be remedied on the spot.

I would repeat this mantra: "You cannot prevent the system from producing errors unless you study the errors that come out of the system."

So we started doing more reviews. No one in Family Medicine would volunteer to be on the quality committee so I put everyone on the committee. A doctor rotated on for four months and then had eight months off.

When we found an error reviewing a doctor's chart that did not harm the patient the doctor would say, "The patient did fine. Why are you bothering me about this?" So it was often better to study the charts of patients who died because even if it looked like the error was not the cause of death (it usually wasn't) nobody could say "Don't bother me, the patient did fine."

I made it my business to learn about as many hospital mistakes or errors as I could. It was not in my job description as Chair. Hospitals don't like to put in writing that they are a place doctors make mistakes, although we live with and catch or miss mistakes every day.

I found a lot of errors over the years, both harmful and "near misses." I tried to utilize many of these errors as learning experiences.

What kind of errors might be made during your medical care? You can divide medical error into errors of omission (forgot to do something) and areas of commission (did something that was wrong for the patient.)

It's not about whether the patient was harmed. If a doctor neglected to treat a low potassium on an otherwise well hospitalized patient it might have resulted in no harm. But if the patient developed a certain type of arrhythmia, affected by low potassium, the patient was clearly harmed by the low potassium.

It was the same error whether the patient was harmed or not.

We should aim to study and learn from these errors. It's not an exercise in "Let's find out who those bad doctors are and we'll get rid of 'em." That wouldn't work because we all make errors. We'd have no doctors or nurses left.

Errors of omission are harder to discover. You are looking for something that's not there.

It's not easy to study error in the medical field because people go out of their way to hide their mistakes. Admitting to a serious error can adversely affect your career whether are a doctor, a nurse, or in a related medical field.

Yes, let me tell you, doctors never write in the chart, "Whoops, I made a mistake."

It's just the opposite. You had to carefully pore over the charts, trying to decipher the bad handwriting and infer what the doctor was thinking day by day. I spent many hours on Sundays studying the work done by my department.

Most of us learn from our own mistakes. We hope so anyway. In my 21 years in leadership, I may have seen more mistakes than a typical doctor would encounter in 200 -300 years of practice. That's a crazy thought!

I confess that made me a lot more cautious in my own practice.

Maybe that slowed me down seeing patients. To learn in a lecture about a spinal abscess as a possible cause of back pain is one thing. It's another matter to study the case of a patient who died when that problem was not found promptly because subtle clues were missed early in the course.

This process requires a delicate touch. No matter how nicely you handle it, finding, and even anonymously discussing errors causes bad feelings in doctors. You will make enemies. I have read in the safety literature that hospital error reduction requires strong support from the CEO and the Board. In my case, I had the support of Dr. Butcher and the hospital risk management people. In retrospect, I cannot believe I did it for so long without enthusiastic backup from the very highest levels of hospital administration.

Trying To Make Finding Error a Good Thing

I tried my best to promote error finding as a good thing.

At the department meeting, I would say something like, "Today, we're going to discuss a serious error discovered by our quality improvement committee. If you were the doctor involved, keep that to yourself. Anyone in this room could have made the same error. What matters is that we learn something from going over this case."

I never met a hospital administrator who was enthusiastic about the search for errors in his or her hospital. I found that hospital administrators are more interested in seeing financial reports. They also love seeing improving numbers on statistics that are collected at the behest of the government and insurance companies. They call these statistics "metrics."

Our hospital risk management people very much appreciated what I was doing. They knew their job was really managing disasters more than managing risk. They liked the idea of fewer disasters. It's better to choose to prevent a disaster than to be forced to deal with one. We say that's being proactive rather than reactive.

To me, a lot of the typical "metrics" being collected in those days were not especially relevant to patients. I think they are better today.

But for the most part, hospitals track **outcome** indicators. Not **process** indicators. If you were a bakery your outcome measurement would be how deliciously the cakes taste. A process indicator could be how accurately the flour was being measured in each cake.

Medical outcome indicators sound great but the favored endpoints are unambiguous measurements like "number of deaths" instead of "quality of life after treatment," which also matters but is harder to measure.

You can't just tell a group of doctors to improve outcomes.

"Ladies and Gentlemen of the Surgery Department, we need a lower post-op infection rate. Get to it!!"

The surgeons will look at each other: "We are the best surgeons we know. What are we supposed to do? Are you attacking us?"

They would do better with process indicators:

To those surgeons: "Your peers on the committee have decided. We're going to work on improving the number of patients who scrub with an antiseptic the night before surgery. We're going to culture up patients who in the past year have had family members with staph infections and hold surgery until they test negative. We're going to observe and measure hand washing practices pre-op and post-op. We're going to implement checklists. We're going to standardize preoperative antibiotics and make sure they conform to guidelines."

Outcome or Process: which is better? Here is an outcome metric: What hospital in our city has the lowest inpatient death rate for heart attack patients? Sounds like a good question. I think I want to go to the hospital with the lowest rate.

OK, maybe so. But what if that hospital with the lowest inpatient death rate for heart attack (an outcome metric) is missing something in the treatment. Let's say we find out that its patients more often die at home within a month after being discharged? Maybe they sent the worst patients home earlier to die there to make their inpatient death statistics look better. If we could look at a different outcome measurement, the death rate *30 days after discharge* maybe we find it was not as good at the hospital we thought was better based on the *inpatient* death rate?

127

Outcome metrics can be messed up. The hospital only wants you to see the outcome stats that make them look better. They are good for comparison and bragging rights.

Outcome metrics can be based on circumstances beyond the hospital's control. What if one hospital has more affluent patients and the other one has patients who average very low income. We know that as economic factors worsen, health statistics get worse too.

You can tell I don't find outcome measurements to be very useful. I remember my CEO once said we had a slightly higher inpatient death rate than the other big hospital in town. We had to take action!

The inpatient death rate statistic sounds very important but it is easily affected by external factors. Some doctors get more of their patients to accept hospice care and those patients tend to die at home. The result is fewer inpatient deaths. Other doctors do just the opposite. I knew some doctors who were so good at keeping hopelessly ill patients alive just a little longer that their patients were admitted again and again over a period of weeks before they finally died. More of those patients died in the hospital.

I asked that CEO who was worried about out inpatient death rate if he knew what the death rate was in the United States. He said he did not. I told him, "It's 100%" That's because everyone dies. He was not happy with me for that quip.

Another type of metric or thing that is measured is called a process metric. In this metric we track how the hospital follows best practices. Keeping with the subject of heart attacks, we can check what percentage of patients with an early heart attack received "clot buster" drugs within thirty minutes of arrival compared with those who received this therapy after 30 minutes? You are now studying how well the hospital team conforms to the best practices. That's the process of care. Getting the clot-buster within thirty minutes is better. The hospital with the better percentage is through-putting the heart attack patients faster. That's good.

Process measurements more directly derive from the study of errors. In other words, when you find where you are making errors or might make errors you study the process where the errors are made.

Here is another case that has been changed just enough to make the identity of the patient undiscoverable. A patient arrives in the ER with a history of chest pain for 48 hours. The triage nurse decides that this has been going on too long to be an acute heart attack.

If the nurse thought the symptom might have been an acute heart attack he/she would jump that patient to the front of the line. You must do that to meet that thirty-minute clotbuster goal.

Unfortunately, it turns out the chest pain had been very, very mild for two days and very severe for the past 15 minutes. It was two days of pre-heart-attack chest pain followed by a massive clot in a coronary artery or a heart attack. That clot needed clot-buster drugs fast. The error was not asking the right questions. The nurse was too rushed. The patients did not get the clot buster drug on time. What can we learn from this case? We can tell all the triage nurses that having chest pain for days before the actual heart attack can happen. We can put that in their policy manual that they must study before taking the triage nurse position.

We acknowledge that the process measurement "percentage of heart attack patients who receive clot-buster treatment within 30 minutes of arrival to Emergency" is very pertinent.

The very important associated outcome measurement is "deaths in heart attack patients." The measurement of treatment in 30 minutes is a critical part of the outcome.

We don't know how to improve our process unless we study each error from every case that went over the 30-minute standard. If we study each case where we failed, we might figure out what in our process needs to change.

In the late 1980's when I was charged with improving the care given by the doctors in my department, we had not established good process or outcome measures.

Some hospital leaders at that time tried to judge their quality by measuring the data they already had in their computers.

They said, "You don't need to roll up your sleeves. You don't need to dirty your hands touching those charts for hours on early Sunday mornings while your family is still sleeping. We have a ton of data in our computers. We can improve quality by studying that stuff. That'll be faster, too."

The electronic medical record had not been implemented. The data they had was billing data. Who got charged for what?

It was like trying to figure out how to make driving safer by analyzing drivers' license data on what city people lived in or whether they lived in a house or an apartment. We could see when a drug was prescribed but we couldn't be sure when or whether it was given to the patient.

Do you want to know how to find the driving mistakes that really matter? Figure out the stuff that drivers would prefer to conceal after accidents.

Like: I was texting before the collision. I was eating. I was speeding. I took a tranquilizer. I had my eyes off the road. I was sleepy.

Investigating bad outcomes can lead to error-finding. Studying errors leads to process analysis and eventually to process improvement. How do we do this part of our work and how can we do it better? Fix the process. That can lead to better outcomes.

Every hospital wants the public to believe its doctors are highly experienced. We have established that experience comes from either studying your own errors or the errors of others. But the hospitals like to pretend errors rarely happen and doctors and nurses learn it's best to hide them. Something's wrong.

That's why I tried to make the discovery of errors a good thing. The things everybody wants to hide are the very thing we need to study so we can fix how we do things. I used to repeat this mantra: **you cannot fix a system that permits errors unless you study the errors that come out of the system.**

I See the Problem!!

It's during the French Revolution, and a line of condemned Frenchmen are waiting for the guillotine. The first man is marched up, hands tied behind his back. They put his neck on the frame where necks go when someone is about to be beheaded. The executioner pushes the button.

The blade comes down two inches and stops.

The executioner exclaims: "Mon Dieu. It's a miracle. French law states that when this happens, it must be the will of God. You are free. You may go."

The second man is marched up. Same procedure. The executioner resets the guillotine. He pushes the button. The blade falls two inches and stops.

The executioner exclaims: "Mon Dieu. Another miracle! French law states that when this happens, it must be the will of God. You are free. You may go."

The third man is marched up. He says, "Hey mister! I think I see what's wrong with your machine."

"Something's Went Wrong. Nobody Say Anything"

Somewhere in life, we have all learned to not speak up when something goes wrong. School kids will say, "Don't be a rat."

But if we are serious about finding errors in our medical workplace, we have to make it normal for front-line people to report them. The big bosses don't know what happens on the front lines: not the Chief of this, or the Vice President of that, or the Director of the other. It's the front-line workers who see the errors. By front-line I mean the people who actually touch patients.

Most mistakes are caught by the person who almost made them. Many errors are caught before anything happens to the patient. Some get through to the patient but the patient is not harmed. Sometimes the patient is harmed, but the harm is minor. Usually, several workers on the front-line team know about those errors the day they happen. Sometimes and it might be rarely, the error is very serious or even fatal. Those cases are usually studied extensively by people in top leadership. And sometimes plaintiff's lawyers get involved.

We don't need to wait for that serious type of error. We can acknowledge that you can learn a lot from the same errors that don't cause harm.

After serving as Chief of Family Medicine, I became Vice President of Medical Affairs. Many doctors who aspire to that position, get a Masters Degree in Business Administration (an MBA). I told people I didn't have an MBA so I had to have an MBWA. That stands for "Management By Walking Around."

Every day I spent an hour walking through every part of the hospital saying hello to people. I did it in the morning. Sometimes I went around at 6 PM. Sometimes on weekends. I became familiar. I wasn't just a name on a memo or a voice on the phone. Sometimes people such as nurses, aids, technicians, and doctors confidentially told me things I needed to know. They told me about care in the hospital.

I knew all the doctors on the medical staff. Some had reputations for complaining a lot. It would have been easy to turn them off. "Can you write me a letter about that? I am late for a meeting."

I didn't do that. I cultivated my complainers. They were the ones who told me what was wrong at the hospital. If it was a nursing issue, I discussed the problem with the director of nursing (DON). I told the DON that I had heard from one of my canaries. I called these doctors canaries

133

because that's the bird coal miners take into the mine. When there's a leak of dangerous gases, the canaries are the first to fall over. They let everyone else know there is a problem.

Canaries don't send letters. They don't send emails. They chirp, they warble, they sing and they chatter. But you have to be near them to hear them.

I recently spoke with an old friend who had been Chief Operating Officer (COO) when I was VPMA. He left our hospital for a big promotion, a job as a hospital CEO. He told me that he brought something to the new job he learned from me, my MBWA or "Management By Walking Around." At his hospital on his orders, no meetings were allowed between 9 and 10 a.m. Every department leader was to use that time to walk around the hospital to visit not just their own departments but to interact with and learn from every other section of the hospital.

I need to confess I didn't invent MBWA. I met a lot of leaders who never heard of it so I talked it up. It's a great way to uncover errors by hearing from people who would never put it in writing.

Errors are common. We should seek the errors we call "near misses." These are the errors that don't lead to the huge lawsuits. We can study those and see if there is something that we can do to error-proof our processes. I will go over near misses a few chapters ahead.

Sleepy Driving and More

I wonder whether traffic accident report forms contain a question about sleepy driving and sleep apnea. The treatment of certain medical conditions and the reduction of traffic deaths are connected. For example, sleep doctors know patients with sleep apnea cause a lot of accidents.

"Excessive daytime sleepiness is a common symptom of obstructive sleep apnea, which can cause you to awaken in the morning feeling tired and unrefreshed despite a full night of sleep," said American Academy of Sleep Medicine President Dr. Timothy Morgenthaler. "Effective identification and treatment of sleep apnea is essential to reduce avoidable, life-threatening accidents caused by drowsy driving."

The AAA Foundation for Traffic Safety estimates that drowsy driving may cause 328,000 motor vehicle accidents and 6,400 fatal crashes on U.S. roads each year. ☼

Source:https://aasm.org/risk-of-motor-vehicle-accidents-is-higher-in-people-with-sleep-apnea/

This danger is known to every primary care doctor and every sleep specialist.

When you first apply for a driver's license they may ask something like "Do you have any visual/medical condition(s) affecting your ability to drive safely? Should the medical questions be more specific?

After an accident would the police investigating the colllision ask: "Have you ever been diagnosed with sleep apnea, or had treatment recommended that you are not following?"

That's not what happens.

I suppose a lot of likely drivers being interviewed after an accident would not answer honestly. Maybe in suspicious circumstances, accident investigators could use the threat of getting the drivers medical records to ferret a more accurate answer to: Did the driver ever refuse a doctor's advice to treat his sleep apnea? Is the driver taking any medication that could lead to enough drowsiness to impair driving?

It is important to point out a diagnostic issue needs to be resolved first. Sleep Apnea is over-diagnosed.☼

In a Swiss study. 50% of men and 23% of women were positive for sleep apnea when tested.

(https://pubmed.ncbi.nlm.nih.gov/25682233/)

In an Icelandic study researchers found about a 20% incidence of Obstructive Sleep Apnea in the general population with no or minimal symptoms.

(https://pubmed.ncbi.nlm.nih.gov/26541533/)

Many of those patients with bonafide symptoms can be treated successfully by being trained to avoid sleeping on their backs. In many cases the snoring and spells of airway obstruction go away on the side. Sadly that treatment approach is not commonly prescribed. More popular with sleep physicians are expensive masks and sleep apnea machines.

I don't ever want the government randomly inspecting my medical records. But with rights like the right to drive comes responsibility. At least we could ask drivers involved in accidents if they suffer from frequent daytime drowsiness.

Currently, we are not adequately screening high-risk drivers with broad, generic questions when they renew their licenses. How's that working? Just for sleep apnea, we find 6400 vehicular deaths a year! I don't think what we are doing is working. "Hey mister, I think I know what's wrong with your machine."

That's only one medical condition. We didn't even talk about seizures. We need self-driving cars that drive better than people do.

My point? I'm against death due to driving errors but my earlier topic was medical errors. There are times when reasonable people keep their mouths shut. They don't volunteer information. They clam up after they make a mistake. They clam up after their friends or colleagues make a mistake. No one wants to "rat out" their colleague.

"It was just a mistake." "It will never happen again, let's not get anyone into trouble."

"He's a good doctor, what a shame, these things happen." "We don't need to file a report."

How can we get around this kind of avoidance of reporting error in the medical field?

If we want to implement a system in which people feel safe reporting errors, we have a lot of work to do. It is easy to implement policies that say error reporting is non-punitive. But such policies don't work unless every level of leadership supports the idea with the highest levels of leadership being the loudest cheerleaders.

Hospital Boards of Trustees need to remove hospital CEOs who don't enthusiastically implement programs of error reporting. CEOs should give an update on that topic at every meeting of the hospital's governing board. It's leadership that takes those policies out of the policy book and makes them work.

Maybe we need to go beyond punishment-free reporting. Maybe we should reward people on the front line who point out our mistakes.

What is the patient's role in all of this? First, you need to know that it is your right to receive medical care with the lowest possible number of errors. Reducing errors that harm has a name. It's called Patient Safety. You also need to know that experts estimate that in well-to-do countries close to 10% of hospitalized patients are harmed by what they call "adverse events," and 50% of those events are preventable. **The result is that medical error is one of the leading causes of death**. ☼

Reader! Are you connected to someone on the Board of Trustees at a hospital? Talk to them. If you volunteer at a hospital you are a VIP. Hospitals treasure their volunteers. Ask to speak to someone and ask about patient safety and error finding. Are you someone who stirs thing up on social media? Then do that. If you have the chance to ask people in authority, ask about what your hospital is doing to reduce error.

Do they seek to uncover errors and then study them?

If you are the patient or the family member of a patient who encounter an error, write a letter!

"I want to point out a problem during my hospital stay. I observed an error in my care. I know that no hospital is perfect but I also know that the best hospitals seek out their errors and learn from them. Here is what happened to me...."

Remember my mantra: *you cannot fix a system that permits errors unless you study the errors that come out of the system.*"

Near-Misses

The best mistakes to study we can call "near-misses."

If a patient is harmed due to an error, doctors know they are required to report the matter to their malpractice insurance carrier.

Defense lawyers get involved and tell everybody to clam up.

Luckily, there are a ton of errors that don't harm. They are caught and corrected before that patient is harmed or due to dumb luck they just don't do noticeable harm. A harmless error can be identical to a fatal error so near-misses are just as good to study. They can be discussed with relative ease if you make the study of errors part of your organization's culture.

So a critical part of fixing the errors permitted by your system is to encourage reporting of near-misses.

This idea was part of how I operated as Chair of my Family Medicine department.

When I identified an error that would be useful to improve how we practiced, it was important to share it with the whole department rather than just the doctors involved. I would present several cases briefly at the monthly department meeting. I would say, "I have a few cases to discuss today. I repeat from an earlier chapter:

"Here are the rules: If *you* were the doctor involved, don't identify yourself. If you know who was the doctor involved, keep that to yourself please. The point of these cases is they involve errors that could be made by anyone in this room. Our subject is the error, not the doctor who made the error."

When a room full of doctors heard about an error at one of those meetings, there were a lot of private "object lessons" being absorbed.

Sometimes one doctor will speak up with an idea on how to prevent the next instance of this error.

I recall one meeting when we reviewed some cases. This issue was the care of a patient admitted for back pain. The physician who had admitted the patient was recognized by his peers as a solid clinician. The reviewer had questioned whether the patient had needed to be admitted.

Now I need to introduce another physician, the one who reviewed the case. This doctor was recognized as very weak clinically. I did not know what to do with him. You can't just say "Everyone knows your knowledge is out-of-date, stop admitting patients to the hospital." Try that and you will have a lawsuit that you will lose. What I did as Chair was make sure he always consulted specialists for everything and I reviewed a ton of his admissions.

This doctor said, "The physical exam does not mention a rectal exam. If the patient had back pain bad enough to be admitted, the attending should have done a rectal exam. What if the back pain were due to prostate cancer?"

Inside my head, cheers and loud applause broke out. My out-of-date doctor made a perfectly valid point. It would have been very sad if the patient was found months later to have prostate cancer spread to the spine. The weakest doctor in the department was reminding his peers how to practice better medicine. Thank goodness the identity of the admitting doctor was concealed.

Meeting "One on One" with a doctor who made an error is much harder.

When you have to tell a doctor he made a mistake, sometimes you keep thinking, "There but for the Grace of God, go I." Sometimes you get a bad reaction from the doctor.

Defensiveness

Depending on the case, sometimes a one-on-one meetings was necessary. During these encounters I would look for three reactions from the doctor, as I had learned from the writings of Donald Berwick, M.D, a medical quality pioneer. As Chief you are there to help the doctor practice better. But the doctor thinks he/she is being personally attacked. Such a doctor may:

1) Dispute the data

2) Shift the blame

3) Shoot the messenger

Dispute the data: the doctor says he disagrees that things happened the way the chart says they did. "He had a normal potassium just four hours before that low one. How come that's not in the chart?" In those days labs might be on a slip of paper scotch-taped to a page in the lab section of the chart and those could get lost.

Shift the blame: "I consulted a cardiologist on that case. To watch the potassium was the cardioligist's job. Of course, I know low potassium causes arrhythmias. I consulted the cardiologist, didn't I?"

Shoot the messenger: "I have had nothing but trouble from you since you became Chief. What do you have against me? I am reporting you to the Vice President of Medical Affairs"

I learned to look for these reactions. They mean the doctor thought he was being attacked. These are defensive moves.

Later, when I was VP of Medical Affairs, I trained six new department chairs and taught them to look for these three reactions.

When this happens you need to reassure the doctor: We're not talking about your worth as a person. We're not talking about your value as a physician. We are talking about one specific error. It could have been anyone who made that error. We're talking, you and I alone, because you know more about this incident than anyone.

Then I'd ask, how do you think such an error could be prevented?

Do you get an idea why a fixation on collecting outcome metrics is not the most productive way to improve the quality of the doctors' or the hospital's performance?

Confessions of a Sightly Misogynistic Past.

Misogynistic might be too strong a word. But I think a lot of men today realize that some attitudes they possessed years ago were not fair to women. The word misogynistic means *strongly* prejudiced against women. We should be opposed to being *slightly* prejudiced against women too! When I got married I thought I was pro-feminist. I was just a beginner. We all learn, hopefully.

At the time I became Chief of the Department of Family Practice, the head of the department was called the "Chairman." That was in the bylaws. It did not seem sexist, that was just the name.

In fact, a woman had just become chairman of the hospital's Board of Trustees. She was the first. I asked her if she was going to keep that designation. She told me that every man who had held the position had been called the "Chairman" and she felt it was important for her to use the same title.

In that year, our department had a young female faculty member.

She was the only woman in the department. She had only finished her residency training a few years earlier. At the department meeting, I was going over the draft of new departmental bylaws which I had been tasked to rewrite.

Our young faculty member insisted we should rename the position in a way not to favor the male gender. It should be "Chairperson."

One of the male doctors objected. He said that even "person" has a "son" in it. Even Chairwoman has a "man" in it.

An 85-year-old retired doctor who still enjoyed coming to the meetings was the oldest member of the department. He stood up and said, "If you take the "man" out of the "woman", all you are left with is woe.

That is how the discussion ended.

This young faculty doctor went on to be in charge of Family Medicine at the local medical school. She was called the Chair. Later she was recruited for the same position, Chair, at a larger medical school and then another medical school after that.

I now realize that she had been right.

When Doctors Want to Cover the Donkey

Definition of Ass.

1: A donkey

2: Something that needs to be covered as in "CYA."

Patients need to understand that doctors are afraid to be wrong. Our training teaches us over and over to protect ourselves from being wrong by ordering more tests and prescriptions. A lot of time, the patient receives more testing or treatment than would be necessary.

In baseball, if you don't swing when you're at bat you're never going to hit the ball. But sometimes you get on base very nicely by just standing. Resist the temptation to swing at the bad pitches. After four of those you get on base with a "base on balls."

Sometimes a doctor will take a thorough history and perform a competent exam and then decide to do nothing. In these circumstances, maybe a doctor's decision to DO NOTHING should be respected. Your doctor may have been trained to always do something but has learned the value of watchful waiting.

Patients expect their doctors to be genteel. We don't like our doctors to use vulgar words. In that spirit we have the expression, "Put the blanket on the donkey." We only explain we mean CYA after we get a blank stare.

On the other hand if you think your doctor is feeling compelled to order a medication or a test, tell him/her you respect the power of doing nothing when it is appropriate. ☼

"Doctor, if you just want to wait and see for now, that's ok with me; you don't need to put a blanket on the donkey."

Communicating: Learn a Few New Words

Without a doubt, native Spanish speakers are the most common non-native English patients. Most Spanish-speaking patients for whom I had the honor of caring had a good command of English. But a doctor will see many patients who speak no English and require the help of interpreters. I have found that these patients will appreciate if the doctor knows even a few words of the patient's tongue. One good word to know is the word for "pain" in the patient's language.

In the early days of my practice, I had a German-speaking patient who spoke only a few words of broken English. She spent part of the year with her family in a city 5 hours to the south. When she was there she saw my medical school classmate whose last name was Weissbrot. She told me his name was Dr. White Bread! If you don't know German and I confess I only know thirty words, weiss means white and brot means bread.

After that, I always referred to him as Dr. Weißbrot and she perked up when she heard me say his name with my best version of the German pronunciation: vice brot.

Even more important than knowing a few words in the patient's language, learn something about the patient's country. I told the students when someone comes from an exotic location you don't know, that night spend a few minutes with Google Earth and get an aerial view of the patient's city of origin. You could learn a lot in 5 minutes.

You can also express validation of the patient's culture by knowing something about their foods.

Once I had a new Arabic patient who told me where she was from and how she had come to America. It just so happens that hummus is a favorite food of mine. I make it from dry chickpeas rather than canned ones. Using dry ones is more authentic.

I told her I liked hummus and she immediately looked shocked. She said, "Hamas is very bad, very bad."

We had confused the mixture of chickpeas, tahini, garlic, and lemon juice with the Palestinian fundamentalist resistance movement. I guess I didn't pronounce it very well.

We straightened that out and laughed about it.

Laughing bonds people. When people trust you, they give a better history and you can do a better job helping them. It's not about business.

The problem with patients not understanding words goes beyond the word gap of the international patient. Many English-speaking patients don't know very common medical terms in English.

Here is my advice for all patients. If you don't know a medical word that you hear a lot, look it up and then write it down 30 times on a blank piece of paper. ☼ Get that word into your vocabulary. When 18 percent of the Gross National Product is medicine, it only makes sense for the citizens to learn more of the terminology. It makes communication with your doctor easier. If you hear ten unfamiliar words when the doctor is trying to get the message across, you may get lost in the middle of the conversation, no matter how much time he/she takes explaining.

It's English but it's Jargon

Definition of Jargon: Special words or expressions used by a particular profession or group which might be difficult for others to understand.

The medical profession is fond of jargon, same as the other professions.

But the medical profession has thousands of these terms, more than any other field. It's a challenge for the patients of doctors who don't try to avoid using medical jargon when talking to them.

One day I was telling a physical therapist about my approach to back pain. I told her I just tell people to wiggle their back all through the day.

Definition courtesy of Google: Wiggle: move or cause to move up and down or from side to side with small movements, synonyms wriggle, twitch, shimmy, joggle, wag, wobble, shake, twist, squirm, writhe.

That sounds like the lyrics to a dance song from the 1960s.

The therapist said, "Dr. Sinsheimer, that therapy is called MOBILIZATION EXERCISE." She continued, "You can't tell people to wiggle. They aren't going to PAY to be told to wiggle."

I told her that was understandable. I didn't want to leave patients unimpressed with my knowledge by using 8th grade vocabulary when 12th-grade vocabulary would do.

So from that time on, I told my back patients to do mobilization exercises, and then I explained that mobilization was physical therapy jargon for wiggling, small motions to keep the back muscles from locking up.

TNT is not Just a TV Network

In 2000 our family hosted an exchange student from Germany. We are still friends with Markus and his family and we have visited them in Germany several times and vice versa.

When we met Markus he spoke fairly good English and he learned even more as the months passed.

One evening, before coming home, I had to stop at the local TV station to do a public service announcement or PSA. This was when I was the part-time Chief of the Family Medicine department at our local hospital. The hospital called on me to do stuff like PSAs.

The TV crew was very nice and as we took several takes of the PSA they told me what a great job I was doing. They asked if I had been on TV before? Yes, I said, I had.

When I got home I told my wife how the TV folks told me I was "a natural." She said they probably told everybody that. Reality affirmed, I agreed.

A few days later, Markus informed me that he had answered the phone when no one was home. He said it was a man from TNT. My wife said, "The TV network? Maybe they saw your PSA spot and they want you to be a TV doctor."

I said I doubted it, but if that were the case, they would call back.

"Plus," I said, "Isn't TNT just the channel where they play old movies?"

When I came home a few days later, Markus told me, "That man from TNT called again. Oh, but I pronounced it wrong, it wasn't TNT, it was AT&T."

My TV career had ended before it started.

Number Needed to Treat/ Number Needed to Test/ Number Needed to Screen

So now that you are focused on TNT and AT&T, I want to tell you about NNT, which stands for "Number Needed to Treat" or "Number Needed to Test."

NNT is a term many patients have not encountered. It is a term that many doctors don't use conversing with patients. NNT is one way to communicate the odds, when numbers are used to make decisions. It's a useful concept.

Patients need to hear more about NNT. ☼

The Number Needed to Test can also be called NNS or Number Needed to Screen if you analyze the efficiency of screening for disease. How many patients need to be treated before one benefits?   How many patients need to be screened before you find the disease for which you are looking?

Let's give some medical and non-medical examples to help you understand this concept.

How many times do we need to run the dishwasher before the dishes are reasonably clean? One time or you need a new one.

With an acutely swollen lower extremity, how many tests for deep venous thrombosis, or blood clots in the lower extremities, need to be done before you find one patient with clots? About two.

How many times do you need to take your car to the mechanic before they figure out that difficult electrical problem? I wish I knew, it seems like a lot. If more than one, it's too many.

How many patients who suffer a complete cardiac arrest for which a defibrillator won't restart the heart, need to be treated additionally with resuscitation drugs before one life is saved? Difficult question: defibrillation or shocking the patient is very effective in the right patient who has

149

ventricular fibrillation or unstable ventricular tachycardia, but almost zero flatline patients are brought back with drugs. Answer: maybe 10, maybe 100.

When you are considering whether to accept a certain treatment or test, ask how many people need to be treated or tested before one is benefited?

OK, you've got the meaning of the terms.

NNT (treat) for Prostate Cancer Screening

In the treatment of prostate cancer, how many people do you need to treat to help one patient? If doctors found a bunch of prostate cancers with the PSA blood test and all the patients get treatment for this cancer, the evidence shows you need to treat about 50 patients before one is actually helped. NNT=50.

The conclusions of the NNT doctor group (thennt.com): in the various prostate screening studies, the overall death rates between screened and treated and the unscreened were the same. No benefit. NNT = a very high number, per this group.

https://www.thennt.com/nnt/psa-test-to-screen-for-prostate-cancer-2/

Let's repeat that first analysis: after treating 50 men for prostate cancer, one will benefit. The other 49 will have chance of dying from the cancer, the same outcome as those who stayed safely at home and were never screened and for that reason never treated.

Low numbers would be better. Like NNT of 2. If you only needed to treat two patients to help one, that would be a lot better.

There's another concept called NNH. The H is for "harmed." How many people need to be exposed to a test and/or treatment before one is harmed significantly?

Let's say one person out of 100 having tonsillectomy gets a major bleed post-op. You would need to treat 100 to (sadly) significantly harm one patient with tonsillectomy. NNH = 100.

Let's say if you do 100 carotid artery angiograms in the usual patients at risk, one patient gets a stroke. NNH =100. High numbers are better for NNH. The angiogram, an invasive test, is how we used to test the carotid arteries. We shoved a catheter from the arm to the neck and sometimes a piece of plaque broke off and caused a stroke. Now due to technological advances, we can get a picture of the carotid blockages with ultrasound. NNH = unknown, maybe thousands. The new test itself is very safe.

Prostate Cancer NNT is harder to understand. Let's say you are about to have surgery for prostate cancer.

You assume the surgery will help you. If you do well and have no evidence of prostate cancer for say, a decade or two, **you give all the credit to the surgeon.**

What's the truth? What the full picture? There are so many studies and the numbers are a little bit different from study to study. But it's evident that a great majority of patients found by screening for prostate cancer with a PSA or any other test won't die of the disease even if never treated. As men age, about 2/3 of them can be found to have some prostate cancer yet the lifetime risk of dying from prostate cancer is only 3% for all men. We really did not need studies to know that a lot of those "cured" with surgery did not need anything done.

Restating that: at age 70, about 70 men in 100 have prostate cancer, but only three are going to die from prostate cancer.

What explains this apparent paradox? The reason is the most common type of prostate cancer grows so slowly that it would not have killed you, even if you never found out you had it. The less common disease grows very quickly and may still kill the patient even if found with an annual screening test.

In most cases you would die from another cause before the prostate cancer did you in. In many cases, if you were never tested for it, you would die from another cause at a ripe old age before you ever knew you had had prostate cancer.

I am not saying that only a very few prostate cancers spread.

About 10 to 15 percent of them do spread. I am just saying that only maybe 3% out of the 70% what have it, die from having prostate cancer.

But following this surgery or radiation therapy, a lot of the men treated are going to have problems with urine leakage and weak erections for the rest of their lives.

Bummer!

We can define "harm" as causing suffering when there is no benefit.

For those who didn't need treatment such as surgery or radiation, the side effects of prostate cancer treatments we shall call "harm." If only we knew which one patient was the one who would benefit from all this testing and treatment and which were among the 49 of 50 who would only be harmed.

But why is this NNH/NNT concept foreign to so many patients? If you are bored now you know why we don't write about it. But this stuff matters. What would you say if 50 customers at the auto dealer had to pay for cars before one of them got to take a car home? What if you went to the bank to change a $100 bill and only one in 50 times you got your change? That's like what we're doing with prostate cancer screening. We sell 50 cures and only one really got a cure. To use the new car analogy, we somehow reassure the

49 who paid for the car but didn't get to take the car home that everything is fine and we actually helped them.

Check out the Harvard School of Public Health article on this subject, entitled. "For many men diagnosed with prostate cancer, the treatment may be worse than the disease"

https://www.hsph.harvard.edu/news/magazine/the-prostate-cancer-predicament/

One more point: I am glossing over some details like that fact that a very small percentage of these cancers are so bad that the patient dies despite their cancers being found by screening. It's hard enough to get this idea across without discussing the fractional exceptions. I also wish to say I am not against patients accepting this high harm, low payoff treatment. I just think they should fully understand the options. And I mean "understand" not just being "told."

A Flight Out West

It was July 4, 1978. I was 28 years old and just married the month before. We took off from a small airport in Ohio heading for Washington State. In ten days, I was going to start my first practice at a clinic in Kennewick, a small town east of the Cascade Mountains.

My plane was a Cherokee 140, a four-seater that could carry four passengers if you didn't overload it by putting the full 50 gallons of gas it could hold in the wings.

In retrospect, one might wonder why a young doctor just starting out needed an airplane. During my residency, I had extra income from moonlighting and used it to take flying lessons. I fell in love with flying. After getting my license, when I was off duty I could go up in my plane and look down on the city. It made everything look small. With your own plane, it was so easy to fly whenever you felt like it. You didn't have to arrive at the airport at your reservation time and you could return the plane whenever you wanted. You only had to pick a day with good weather, or at least find a day with a few hours of good weather.

And if you bought a plane of the right age, you could sell it for the same price or more a few years later. It did not seem like a foolish hobby.

Six days earlier, the moving van had lumbered off with all our possessions: a mattress, a bureau, a couch, a table and some chairs, some dishes, some clothing, several boxes of books, and all my notes from medical school which I never looked at again. June 30 had been the last day of my Family Medicine residency. After 5 p.m., having faithfully served the final hours of my residency, we were driven by our friends to the Akron Muni airport where my plane was tied down. We flew east to Youngstown, a thirty-minute trip, where my bride's parents lived. We planned to spend the night. That evening, I checked the weather reports. They weren't good.

154

In our part of the Midwest, the weather nearly always comes from the west.

The wind typically comes from that direction too. If you fly west, you fly against the wind. At the typical flying altitudes, the winds blow faster than on the ground. On a day you feel a 5 mph breeze on the ground you might have a 20 mph wind at 5000 feet, and your 120 mph airplane might only be making a ground speed of 100 mph. So a 2400-mile trip to the west could take 24 flying hours or more. But if you start flying west on a Monday morning towards the bad weather for eight hours, you might be running into a storm that's been spending all day heading for you. You'll run into it that afternoon, even though that storm wouldn't have arrived back home until the next day. Flying west often means flying into trouble, weather-wise.

It was for those reasons that I had allowed ten days for the trip.

There were other problems with my plan.

For one, I could only fly VFR or visual flight rules. That meant I could not fly through clouds. I could only fly in good weather. My old $8,000 airplane had limited climbing ability, especially at higher altitudes. We faced mountain passes ahead. When we reached them, the ground itself would be 8000 feet above sea level and I'd be 1000 feet above the ground. My altimeter would read 9000 feet above sea level, near the upper limit of where the little plane could fly. If the thin air up there were hot, it would be worse. What we needed for the mountainous final leg of the trip was a cool, windless day with blue skies.

Some VFR pilots install a very useful device called a wing leveler which keeps your wings level while you study the map. I had a wing leveler too. I had just married her.

On July 1, the weather in Youngstown was just as unflyable as the forecast suggested it would be. We watched TV. On July 2 it was the same. Ditto July 3.

By July 4, I was getting restless. The pilot reports for northern Ohio described a 1000-foot ceiling but without rain. Indiana was good. The one thing in our favor was we were heading towards better weather.

My plane had no radar or the other equipment needed for flying on instruments and I was not licensed to do that anyway. Flying beneath a 1000-foot ceiling when you can't enter the clouds means you climb up to the bottom of the cloud deck and hang there. You would have only 1000 feet between you and the ground. A thousand feet of clear air is the absolute minimum allowance for VFR flight.

With a sense of optimism eclipsing any thought of caution, we took off around 1 PM. Within a few minutes, we were just below the overcast. Unfortunately, we were too low for the radio navigation aids to reach any of the VOR stations (Very High Frequency Omni-Directional Range navigational aids) that usually would have guided us. But I had a plan B. I followed the Ohio Turnpike which headed due west. After an hour or so I saw the toll booth crossing all the lanes indicating the Indiana border. I saw the clouds were separating and in a few minutes, they were gone.

We flew in a conventional manner and at a conventional altitude across northern Indiana. We were tuned to the VOR stations but didn't need them much. It was a beautiful, clear day. Soon we could see the Chicago metro area and the lakeshore. We went well south of Chicago, giving its busy airports a wide berth. Then we flew straight northwest to Rockford, Illinois, where we landed and found a motel. We were 440 miles from our origin. That night we watched the local fireworks from our motel balcony.

I had been calling the flight weather service. More bad weather was coming. Planning this trip for months, I had been hoping for a dry July. Our wishes for good weather were ignored by the weathermen. If wishes were horses, beggars would be riders.

We had to leave early on July 5. I had hoped to make it to Yankton, South Dakota but the weather came upon us too quickly and we had to land in Des Moines, Iowa while it was still safe to fly. We had only flown a few hours.

I recall my conversation with Approach Control at the Des Moines Airport. They saw me on radar but I wasn't sure where the airport was. We were over the city and my wing leveler was helping watch out for other planes. The map was not unfolded on my lap, so I asked for directions to the airport. The air traffic controller asked "5954U, do you see the capital?" I said, "Is that the building with the gold dome?" "Affirmative." I must have been the only person in the entire state of Iowa who would have needed to ask that question. The gold dome was five miles from the airport and they guided me in.

It was less than 24 hours since we had left Ohio and I thought we were making pretty good progress after all. A car could have made it to Des Moines in ten hours but pilots don't think that way.

We found a motel across the street from the airport. I had hoped to make it to Rapid City, South Dakota the next day, a further 515 miles. The Des Moines Flight Service Station or FSS was right across the street. So I walked over a few times a day. In those days you could walk right in and get your weather report in person.

On July 6 the weather was unflyable. On the morning of July 7, it looked fair. Des Moines was OK; Rapid City was OK; Yankton, SD, my alternate airport was OK. But I knew that the storms from the night before had left behind a lot of white cloud debris that would need to be burned off by the warmth of the sun.

We took off from Des Moines around 9 AM. Air Traffic must have remembered me. They gave me a flight path straight out of town. Soon there was a solid but thin undercast below our plane.

I should explain. An overcast is a layer of clouds over you. An undercast is a layer below you. Because this undercast was thin I could still make out the roads and fields below, through the clouds. A thin undercast did not scare me.

Soon, however, the undercast thickened. Looking below, I could no longer make out the ground. I radioed FSS and learned that my destination and my alternate both had good weather. We just needed to get there.

Then an overcast developed. Like the undercast, it started off thin but soon we were the only plane flying between two opaque cloud layers in a beautifully clear zone about a mile high with clear sky ahead. We felt impossibly small and alone but it was beautiful.

My wing leveler held the plane while I reviewed the maps. I radioed FSS again. The weather was still OK at the destination and alternate.

Soon we ran into a bad problem. The blue sky ahead had turned into white. We were heading for a cloud bank. It was maybe ten miles ahead and we would be there in five minutes. We saw white clouds above, below, and ahead.

I looked around and found a hole below in the undercast. That hole was my way out of that mess. I descended, flying slow circles. I would have to dive through that hole in the undercast to be safe and remain legal.

Soon we were at the hole and I descended through it. It wasn't quite large enough and we were "in the soup" for about 15 seconds which seemed an eternity. Suddenly we broke through. I was shocked. We were only about 400 feet above the rolling farmlands of western Iowa.

No panic. I had been trained for this moment. The first task was to look for high-tension power lines. The wings of small planes don't like them one bit. I saw none. Maybe a quarter-mile away I saw a cropduster doing his morning work. That made me feel a little less alone.

I told my wife we had to land. Probably on a level stretch of road. But the roads were all hilly. "You are not landing here!" she commanded. I agreed.

The air was bouncy being so close to those gentle hills so we bounced. We were far too low to know exactly where we were. Our altitude was too low to reach the VORs or FSS. But the plane's compass told me which direction was west and I knew Yankton had been clear so I kept heading west, all the while looking for power lines.

After about thirty minutes we had clear skies again. I climbed to a normal flying altitude and was able to connect to the navigation signals. I checked FSS for the weather at Rapid City. It wasn't perfect.

We were about 150 miles past Yankton when I realized I really didn't feel very well. I felt shaky. I felt exhausted. I felt an overwhelming desire to land. I had been flying for hours. I told my wife we had to find an airport.

I knew we had crossed the Missouri River and were over farms. I saw a smudge on the horizon just over my left wing. I said, "I think that smudge is a town." I banked towards it. In less than 10 minutes we could see it was a very small town. I could see they had an airport to the northeast. A single airstrip.

To determine which way to land, I radioed the airport on the standard frequency but no one answered. I established a normal landing pattern: downwind, base leg, final approach. I came in for a landing. I couldn't land. The runway seemed too short. At first couldn't understand what was wrong. I tried again. I failed again. This time I saw the little wind sock. The wind was at my back. I was trying to land the wrong way. I did a 180 and set up a final approach into the wind which made for an easy landing.

I taxied up to the lone hanger. We saw a young man there working on a plane. I asked him where I was. He said we were in Winner, South Dakota.

We tied down the plane. The young man told me there was one motel in the town, owned by the chiropractor who was himself a pilot and the only doctor in the town. We called the motel. Someone came and picked us up.

The chiropractor was very nice. He took us to dinner. When he learned I was a family doctor headed out to my first practice, he tried his best to sell me on changing my plans and staying in Winner to open my practice there.

I gazed across the table and saw the look of fear in my wife's eyes. She had had misgivings about moving to a small city like Kennewick, a town of 30,000. Winner had about 2000 people. I told him that I had promised myself to the clinic in Kennewick. We went to bed early July 7.

July 8 brought more bad weather. More of the same rolled in on July 9. I was facing the most difficult and dangerous part of the journey, the mountain passes in northern Wyoming. I kept thinking how those passes had an 8000-foot floor. At that altitude, my plane could climb at only 100 feet per second and less than that on a hot day. I knew in my little Cherokee, those passes had to be traversed on a cool, sunny, windless day. A firm breeze blowing over a hill would set off a downdraft that might exceed the plane's climbing speed. That would knock us to the ground. I had this image in my mind of my little Cherokee flying between two huge mountain cliffs barely above the cars on the road below. The weather would have had to be perfect.

160

I threw in the towel. The young man who had been tinkering at the airport agreed to fly the plane from Winner to Kennewick as soon as the weather was OK for the flight. He appreciated the opportunity to log the hours and get the experience. I said I'd pay for the gas and his flight home.

The chiropractor flew us to Pierre, South Dakota in my plane and we caught a commercial flight to Kennewick.

It was late on July 10 and we were at our destination as planned. The moving van had beaten us to the apartment so we were greeted by all our stuff. After a few days of unpacking, I saw my first patient. About six weeks later, the young pilot called. He had safely landed at our local airport. I picked him up.

I only flew my plane about three hours more after that time. Flying was a little too thrilling.

When my wife was expecting our first child, I decided I would quit flying for good. I sold 5954U for $11,000.

Time passed. We left Washington for Ohio after our first child was born, to be closer to family. Four kids came along and grew up. In 2009 we moved to Arizona.

About 32 years after our adventure in the skies, I was in Prescott, Arizona in the locker room of the YMCA after a swim. I heard a guy talking to his friends and I heard him mention Winner, South Dakota. He was about 20 years younger than me. I asked him:

"Did you say something about Winner?"

He said, "Yes that's where I'm from. My father was the town chiropractor."

What is it that makes young men take risks? From what restlessness springs the need for adventures like this one?

As a physician, I learned the sad math of risk-taking. If a proposed course of action (such as trying to fly a plane VFR across the country) has a 1% chance of disaster, and over the course of your life, you make other decisions that also

161

have a 1% risk of disaster, after 100 such risky choices, the odds of a disaster befalling you are 100%. Taking a 1% risk with a patient was something I would not tolerate. There were to be no more 1% risk adventures in my private life either.

Recently at a family gathering, I looked out and saw my four children, their spouses, and my five grandchildren. If my wife and I had crashed and perished on that flight...things would be very different.

Now I'm retired and if I feel the need to take my life into my hands I just walk down the stairs without holding onto the rail. That's a joke, I wouldn't do that.

If I get the urge to fly, I might use a flight simulator computer program. Using my computer and my imagination, once I flew a P-51 Mustang upside-down over the whole length of the runway at Cleveland's airport. My head was only five feet above the simulated pavement. I did not "crash" but it made me nauseated. It's much safer to fly little planes with a simulator program but you still might toss your cookies.

The Three Step Exercise Program

Why do so few people exercise?

In our town, we have a ton of bike paths. They are used by walkers, joggers, and bikers. I'd say you see ten walkers for every jogger. Naturally in the winter, you see nearly no bikers. In my experience, joggers are more prone to injuries than walkers. I can say you rarely see a jogger who looks over 60 years old. I'm not talking about the 50-year-old joggers who look old due to the painful expression on their faces.

Walking is a very natural exercise. I mainly swim but decided to start walking a few years ago and eventually I could go three miles without much fuss.

I recall the expression, "When the spring comes, the saps start running." Just kidding runners, no disrespect intended. Just watch your ankles.

Regardless of walking v running v jogging v biking v swimming: most people are inactive. When I was in practice I always urged inactive patients to do something.

One of my patients shared with me "The Three-Step Exercise Program." ☼

Step One: Schedule when you are going to do it.

Step Two: At the appointed time, put on your exercise clothes.

Step Three: Do it.

The idea is that you feel stupid if you do Step One and Step Two and then just stand around in your exercise outfit staring at the walls.

Exercise relieves stress. I sometimes think about prehistoric man in contrast to modern man.

When prehistoric man had stress, I imagine it usually involved physical danger and his stress was accompanied by some exertion like climbing a tree to get away from some critter with big teeth. But modern man has stress without physical exertion. That's not good.

When someone says something stupid or nasty or you see something which gets you very riled up, where are you? Not climbing a tree. You're probably in front of your computer screen or the TV.

I once heard a lady say, "At times like these, I silently say to myself 'What the f..!!?'" Her friend said, "You're not supposed to say that out loud?"

I think that once you get in shape, with the calm that comes from exercises, you get that Teflon coating that allows those stressors to just slide right off you.

That workout gives your life the balance between stress and exertion. ☼

See the chapter on "The Magic Wallet."

Then why do people remain inactive?

I recall another expression: "*If you knew how to put common sense into common practice, they would ask you to take over the world.*"

Becoming Angry With Patients

Getting angry about things is a waste of energy. During the years I did not exercise, I tried to avoid anger. Like many people, I wasn't always successful at controlling an emotional response. That got easier after I started swimming again at age 43. But once I was hoarse for two weeks after yelling at the dog.

I told patients that you really cannot control how you react emotionally about something. That's just spontaneous. What you can control is how you behave when you are angry. Behaving like a scary person is not my style.

I took care of a couple once who I liked a lot and I knew they liked me. One day I learned from his wife that her husband had transferred to an internist.

She told me why. It was her idea. "My husband likes you but you don't frighten him. That's why he doesn't take better care of his diabetes. I thought that a six-foot, six-inch internist would frighten him into being a better patient. That's why we had his records transferred there."

Later, she told me this plan actually worked. For six months. Then he went back to his old ways.

Despite trying to be calm in a professional way, when you care for patients, things will happen that make you angry, even at them.

I remember a patient who had to be placed on warfarin, an anticoagulant.

Warfarin can be dangerous, because it can cause uncontrolled bleeding, usually when too much is taken.

We compare certain drugs to a two-edged sword. That's an antique weapon from the days of hand-to-hand sword fighting. A heavy sword with both edges sharpened was handy because you could swing the thing back and forth to hit both the guy on your left and the guy on your right without having to rotate the blade. But it could bounce back on you and then you are cut by your own sword. A two-edged sword is effective but dangerous.

Likewise, warfarin could save you from a blood clot but it can also kill you, with an internal hemorrhage or a brain hemorrhage. To avoid that possibilities, we monitor and adjust the dosage of the warfarin with a test called a "Pro-time/ INR."

The patient was a nice fellow but he had the maturity of a 12-year-old. He would not go for his anticoagulation monitoring pro-time at the frequency I advised. He came into the office one day and I learned he had not been to the lab for three months. I had seen patients who nearly died from this type of neglect, and when I criticized him for not going to the lab he made a joke about it.

I was so frustrated that I got angry and I raised the volume of my voice. I remember saying something like, "I'll be damned if you're going to show up dead on arrival at the emergency room with MY NAME on your warfarin bottle."

In retrospect, that was a bit narcissistic on my part.

When I left the exam room I noticed that everybody in my little office was very quiet. No one in the waiting area was saying a word. My staff were whispering. The patient in the next exam room asked me if everything were all right. Apparently, my loud rebuke was heard throughout the entire office.

I hoped the patient would do better and I must say I was delighted when he showed up for his pro-time test regularly for about three months. He then went back to his old bad habits. But soon thereafter I was able to safely stop the warfarin before anything bad happened to him from his self-neglect.

Don't Assume an Incentive Works in Your Favor

Every person who serves the public will earn the admiration of some and the condemnation of others. It should be the ratio of the unhappy to the total number of customers that should count. But we tend to let the experience of a few negative online reviews influence our opinion more than a lot of positive reviews. You cannot learn the true picture from the experiences of just one or two negative-minded persons.

People work better with the *right* incentives. You need to step into someone's shoes to effectively judge if the incentives that you thought were going to favor your interests are going to be effective.

For visits to the doctors' office, the longer, more complex visits are paid more. That's a good incentive for complicated patients, right? The doctor will want to spend the extra time.

Not really. Although the fee schedule pays more for complexity, if you look at the time equivalents of those different classes of visits, the pay per minute goes way down with the longer ones. Fast, superficial medical care pays a lot better, per minute.

Real estate commission are interesting. We all know stories of realtors who disappointed the customer selling a home. You would think that being paid by commission would incentivize the maximum effort to get a great price. But when you think about it, the fact that they receive a commission based on the sales price does not guarantee a full effort for the top price.

Wait a minute: the higher the sales price, the more the realtor gets, right? True... but.

You are selling your home. You reject an offer and tell your realtor you want to get $5,000 more. It's more efficient for the realtor to urge you to take the current offer and move the sale along. At a commission of 7.5% of the selling price your realtor might only see 1/4 of that because she has to split the commission with the buyer's broker and then her brokerage company will take half of what's left. So, she ends up with only 25% of 7.5% = 1.88%. If the buyer agrees to the higher price, what does the realtor get? Answer: their extra 1.88% of your "let's wait to get an extra $5,000" is only $94 in the realtor's pocket, and that's before taxes.

From the realtor's viewpoint, it's much better to sell your house for the first respectable price offered, the one lower than you wanted, and hold onto the hope that a reputation for a fast sale brings in more new customers than building a reputation for getting top dollar.

The incentives in running a doctor's office are interesting too. Twenty years ago we drove through San Luis Obispo, California. I thought it would be a hoot to swim in their community pool because it's called "Sinsheimer Pool." Although my last name is unusual, in this town they have had a lot of Sinsheimers.

A school, a park, and a pool are named after Louis Sinsheimer who served as mayor from 1919 to 1939. The late Dr. Robert L. Sinsheimer, PhD, the father of the human genome, not my relation, also came from that town.

Our rental car got a flat tire in the pool's parking lot. I was changing it when a swimmer came out of the pool and offered to help us. We chatted. He told us he managed the office of his wife who was a family doctor. I asked if it were true that running a private practice in California was difficult as I had read.

He said something like, "Not if you know how."

I asked him what that meant and he told me something like this: "The most important thing is to make the right

168

appointments. If someone calls and says they're not sure if they are sick enough to come in, *bring them in!!* If someone calls and says they are very sick, *send them to the ER.* The patient you want is the one the doctor can see quickly. The complicated ones mess up your schedule and you lose money on them."

My youngest daughter who was about 14 was appalled to hear this. Today she has her Master's Degree in Hospital Administration and ethics rule her worldview.

As I said, don't assume the incentives in place work in your favor. See the chapter called "Never Expect Someone to Make a Change in Their Life Unless You Give Them an Adequate Reason To Do So." That applies to the motivation of doctors and medical centers, not just the motivation of patients.

Promises

I heard about a politician who went to a town in the most rural corner of the state to seek votes for the upcoming election. The town leaders told him, "What we really need here is a family doctor." The politician whipped out his cell phone and dialed a number. He excused himself as he talked for a few minutes on the phone and then announced, "You'll have a family doctor here within a year!" Then the town leaders said, "The other thing we desperately need here is some cell phone reception."

Family Medicine, the In-Demand Specialty

I just read that the medical specialty in the highest demand is Family Practice. Yet our average pay is on the lower end of the spectrum for doctors. How's that supposed to incentivize students to go into Family Medicine?

I am not complaining about what I earned as a doctor. But as a young doctor, it was a bit painful for me to learn that a couple who both worked on the GM assembly line earned more than I did and with better benefits. When you put down this book to Google what Family Doctors earn, realize that half the doctors make less than the average and it can be a lot less.

In my medical school in Cincinnati, we were encouraged to go into a sub-specialty. It was only the rebels in the class who entered residency training in that new thing called Family Practice, which had been reborn from the ashes of General Practice. Exactly 10% of our medical school class went into Family Practice. All were pioneers.

When I was practicing in northeastern Ohio, the state opened a new medical school explicitly to train more family doctors. They did everything possible to encourage their students to apply to Residency in Family Medicine after graduation. Less than a decade after I had entered Family Medicine training, I found out that at this school, now known as NEOMED, just 10% of the graduates went into Family Medicine. The rate was just the same as in Cincinnati where Family Practice had been discouraged.

My residency director, the late John Schlemmer MD, was a model physician. He was smart and altruistic and he had a sense of humor. His program was in high demand. I was one of four chosen out of about 70 applicants.

In those days when you went to a hospital case conference, in many presentations they would explain how the sick patient came to the wondrous medical center after being mismanaged or misdiagnosed by the LMD which stood for "Local Medical Doctor." Dr. Schlemmer humorously referred to his medical school as the place where he received his "LMD."

We are to believe that Family Practice offers lower pay, lower prestige, and yet higher demand? The dollar loaf of bread would be in high demand too. What comes out of a system is the result of how the system was designed. Our medical education system has not been designed to produce Family Doctors. Our fees for Family Medicine services do not compete with what can be earned in many other specialties.

In this book I encourage you to get your physician to spend more time with you when required for shared decision-making and complex diagnostic problems. I want you to realize that the monetary remuneration is not there to incentivize practice that way.

If you are a premedical student reading this book, don't be discouraged by the prospect of lower "monetary remuneration." If you go into family practice, or similar primary care specialties you may not be able to join the country club or drive the fanciest cars but you might just sleep better at night. I used to tell my medical students, family medicine is at the top of the scale for "non-monetary" remuneration.

Watch the Language

Watch carefully how words are used. English can be tricky. For example, a lot of people don't consider the meaning of ads that say, "Up to 70% off!!!" I don't think advertisers would use this pitch if enough people knew that means "Only 1% off is within the range of 'up to 70%' off."

Or up to 70% off could mean, "There is one product in this store that is 70% off."

Words! In Lewis Carroll's <u>Alice in Wonderland</u>, we find Alice talking to Humpty Dumpty.

"When I use a word," Humpty Dumpty said in rather a scornful tone, "it means just what I choose it to mean — neither more nor less."

I remember about 35 years ago when my wife and I were discussing how to clean the kitchen floor. I proposed using a wet mop followed by a wet-dry vacuum with a squeegee attachment would pick up the dirty water. That was a weird idea in 1988. Now our floor cleaning machine does the same thing. It puts down clean, soapy water on the floor and immediately sucks up dirty water. Anyway, in 1988 I thought my idea would be faster and easier. But that wasn't how normal people like my wife cleaned the floor those days. They used a bucket and a sponge. Get down on the floor and scrub. Wring the sponge into the bucket. Repeat.

She said, "If you don't get on your knees, you CAN'T see the dirt."

I said, "That's my point. If you don't get on your knees, you can't SEE the dirt."

Words can have dual meanings. Years ago we almost sold our house on our own without listing it with a realtor. A couple came to our open house and showed interest but never followed up. A realtor contacted us with an attractive offer, "We have a buyer for your home if you sign with us."

We should have thought to ourselves, "What? This buyer wants our house but won't buy unless this particular realtor gets the commission?"

We should have spotted something fishy.

Technically, what that realtor said was not a lie. His firm did have a buyer for the house. They had a customer who they talked into viewing the house, a customer who was not interested in our type of house, but who was a warm, air-breathing person. We later learned that from the realtor's viewpoint there are only two types of people on this entire planet: Buyers or Sellers. And if you are not a Seller, you are a Buyer. So when they said they had a buyer for the house, it might have meant "We have a completely random person who we have asked to look at your house."

Happily, they did find a REAL buyer after about a month. We knew the people. It was the same couple who almost bought it when we were selling it on our own a month earlier.

We should have stipulated in the contract that there would have been a 50% reduction in the commission if the eventual buyer had been someone who visited one of our Open Houses when we were selling on or own. Live and learn.

Words. When you hear outlandish claims, common with health supplements and the like, fly the caution flag. If it's too good to be true or if only this one guy/gal knows the answer to your problem, you should smell that something is not right. In the United States, it's legal to lie about a supplement in a magazine but the FDA says you can't lie on the label. ☼ See if they're willing to risk going to jail by putting a lie on the bottle.

Listen to the claims for prescription drugs too. The drug might lower your blood sugar or your Hemoglobin A1c, but does it lower it enough to make a difference? A drug or treatment can be called effective even if it only helps one person in twenty or more. Listen to the words they use. Are they potentially accurate but deceptive? Is it like "up to 70% off?"

Everything I'm telling here is common sense but a lot of people never figure this out.

Good Deeds. God's Deeds.

I have talked to patients who were Roman Catholics, Protestants, Evangelical Christians, Sikhs, Buddhists, Hindus, Muslim, and one who was a Native American Minister and all agreed with this idea:

God can do anything but prefers to do things with His mind. He wants people to do the things that require hands.

We see too many people these days who confuse "thinking" the right thing or "believing" the right thing with doing the right thing. They think God is contented with thoughts and prayers alone. If that's what they believe, I don't buy it.

Likewise people feel guilty for thinking the wrong thoughts. I have never believed that you can prevent a thought from coming into your head. That thought was residing somewhere in a deep part of your brain, the unconscious part which you are not able to control. Freud originally called it the subconscious mind. The deep brain shoots that thought over to the conscious part of your brain, the part where you can hear your thoughts. You cannot stop it. You can't control your unconscious brain, it's more powerful than the conscious.

What counts should be behaviors not thoughts.

If patients who I counseled seemed to have trouble distinguishing thoughts from behavior, I would tell them: If you can videotape it, it's a behavior. If you can't, it's probably a thought.

Some people are like the wrong kind of churchgoers, who come to church, pray fervently, sing loudly and then go home and don't practice good deeds. Think of Michael Corleone in Godfather I, who is praying in church at his son's baptism as his henchmen are carrying out his plan to murder the leaders of the other families.

Some people are like sports-fans who only watch the game. They wear the team hat and the official sweatshirt. But they are not out there on the field. They are not playing with the team. In life they root for good deed doers, they just don't do many good deeds themselves.

On TV we see earthquake survivors helping search for buried victims after an earthquake. The survivors don't gather around and think nice thoughts about the people buried under the rubble, do they? No, they get in there and dig with their hands.

I've heard a theory that the survival of human society depends upon people helping each other. It's pretty obvious really. Society would not exist if we all just went out on our own like those few solitary members of the animal kingdom.

The list of solitary animals includes some really weird creatures. Wolverines, sea turtles, honey badgers, frogs, armadillos, sloths, Tasmanian devils, giant anteaters, koalas, orangutans, moles, and platypuses prefer to be on their own and only get together with others when it's time to mate.

What makes us want to help others? According to one hypothesis the brain produces a chemical that makes you feel good when you help someone.☼ With regular exposure, this feel-good chemical can become addictive.

We know that athletes will produce endorphins which are pain relieving and feel-good chemicals but the exact feel-good chemical from helping others hasn't been identified by chemists.

So if God decided He would make things with His brain and He wanted people to do the things that require hands, it would have been really smart of Him to create this chemical for our brains.

Good deeds lead to good feelings. Good feelings lead to good deeds. More good deeds produce more good feelings.

175

More good feelings produce more good deeds. It's called a virtuous cycle (the opposite of a vicious one)

There is a problem with this concept of a positive feedback loop of good deeds causing good feelings. How does the cycle get started? What prompts the first good deed?

Maybe that's divine inspiration. Or it could be empirical self-interest. Or the empiricism could have been divinely inspired.

In my experience you have to push yourself to get started. Or permit yourself to be pushed. So sometimes when you're not happy, maybe you need a happiness drug: the happiness drug that comes from helping your fellow man. Start by being nice to people.

When you retire, sign up for volunteer work. Look for opportunities. Push yourself.

A Fast-growing Cancer and the Perfect Teapot

Years ago I had a very nice patient who was a welder. He was 10 years into the age of retirement and still worked part-time jobs because his skill was in demand. He lived modestly. I helped him through some difficult times including the death of his spouse.

One day he presented with a symptom that required testing. In short order, I discovered that he had widespread metastatic cancer.

That you are dying of cancer is always the most difficult thing a doctor has to tell a patient. The tumors were spreading quickly. He was losing weight and strength. We both knew he was dying. He said he felt like he was falling apart.

We had several visits after that as he rapidly deteriorated despite treatment from the oncologists. The tumors were growing too fast.

In a case like this, it's hard to know how to help the patient but a good policy is to sit down and listen to what they have to say. One day he felt compelled to tell me this story which I will never forget.

It was a story about a teapot told in a way that a welder might tell it. He described the construction of a teapot. A lot of parts have to be fabricated and then welded together. There's the main body where the tea is brewed. Below that are the feet which elevate the body off the table to protect it from the heat. The handle is welded to the body as is the spout. Then there's also the lid with a knob at the top. Sometimes there's a filter built into the spout to keep the tea leaves from going into your cup. That is yet one more part that can break.

My patient explained that anytime a weld is created it can break over time. The more welds, the greater the odds

177

that one will fail. If the spout fails the teapot's life is over. If the handle fails it's the same. In fact, if any of the many welds fail, the teapot is no longer of use.

Hundreds of years ago a craftsman built a marvelous teapot. It was so excellently welded that it lasted and lasted. All the welds held. This teapot was as perfect as man can make something. It was passed down from generation to generation until it was over 1000 years old. It was used every day by each family that inherited it.

But God knows that nothing can last forever, even a perfectly made teapot. Tears welled up in my patient's eyes as he told me the rest of the story.

One day the owner opened the door of the cabinet to get the teapot out. There was nothing to be seen but a pile of metal scraps. All the welds had failed at the same time.

By this time my patient was smiling but his voice was breaking. I must confess that my eyes were filling with moisture too. I knew exactly what he meant by the story.

He felt blessed by his life; and he felt that he was like the perfect teapot which sadly could not last forever. It was natural to simply fall apart, all at once.

He had found a way to cope with the end of his life, the metastatic cancer, and the quick deterioration. He accepted it. He was thankful for being "well-made," and for having had a good life. He thought that this way of dying was actually fitting.

A Painless Doctor Fixes a Star-shaped Laceration

We all like praise and thank yous. As time passed I learned the highest compliment a patient can pay the doctor is getting better. I think that is because with experience we learn we would rather see good news from the patient than receive words of praise. I'll explain that.

I still remember the first patient in medical school who paid me a huge compliment. It was during my suture room assignment.

The dreaded suture room! During our third year of medical school, everyone in the class was assigned a 24-hour solo shift in the Emergency Department suture room. The key word is "solo." That meant each of us was the only person assigned to suture up just about every laceration that came in for 24 hours. Before this dreaded day, most students had never sutured a laceration for a real patient. We had sewed pigskin in a classroom. No, not live pigs, just the skin.

We started our shift awkwardly and slowly with a resident physician looking over every suture and by the end of the 24 hours we finished experienced and confident. No sleep was expected and none was to be had. But that was OK because we knew we would get this difficult duty only one time in our medical school careers.

It was my day in the suture room. It was 3 a.m., and I had four hours to go. I was tired. I had closed more lacerations than I could remember but I must say I remember some of those cases to this day, 50 or so years later.

A man who had been drinking too much that evening was brought in with a jagged, star-shaped laceration of the forehead. He had fallen as in the expression "Falling down drunk."

179

I could deduce from other scars on his face that this wasn't the first time he had suffered this type of injury. As I cleaned the wound I recognized it was a difficult case. I calculated how I could put the skin back together, building on what I had learned from the simpler cases I had done in the preceding 20 hours. I anesthetized the edges of the wound and began to work. I placed the sutures so that none would be too tight. Too much pressure in the tissue from a badly placed suture could cause the wound edge to die. I was careful to keep the edges even. Otherwise the skin would buckle. After about 20 minutes the wound was closed; my sutures brought the edges together evenly without being too tight.

The whole while, the patient kept saying he couldn't believe how well I was doing. I guessed the local anesthesia worked perfectly because he kept saying he couldn't feel a thing, nothing hurt. Finally he said, "You know, you're a painless doctor." It was the biggest compliment I had received in my short career of caring for patients.

I told the supervising resident about the case. "I'm a painless doctor," I said. The resident said, "I know that fellow. He's here a lot. He wouldn't have felt anything if you'd forgotten to anesthetize the wound. That guy was three sheets to the wind."

That's why good results count more than high praise.

Towards the end of my career, I was asked: "As a doctor, what is the most unusual way a patient has thanked you for taking care of them?"

I am sorry to say but I can't remember anything really unusual. Sure, people have baked me something, or given me a jar of home-prepared relish, or sent a nice card. One dear patient brought me a jar of spicy, hot horseradish to every visit until finally, he brought me a sprig of the plant and I started growing it on my own.

The best thank you, the one I always appreciated the most, was seeing the patient get better. And a patient who reminded me of how I had once helped them gave me a little energy boost that lasted the day.

By contrast, I remember a patient who never thanked me. She came in one day for something else and I found a large pulsating abdominal aneurysm that needed surgery right away. Aneurysms that large can suddenly rupture and result in death in an hour or two. Often they cause no symptoms beforehand. I sent her to a surgeon and he fixed it. A horrible, painful, aneurysm rupture had been prevented. Her life had been saved.

A year after that she came in with wax in her ear and in the process of removing it, I accidentally caused a small perforation of her eardrum. When you irrigate an ear canal, you can only see the side of the wax ball that faces you. Her wax must have had a sharp edge to it on the hidden side close to the eardrum.

I knew right away I had caused a small perforation and so I sent her to a specialist. He supervised her recovery which was not difficult.

For years after that, she would remind me of the time I put a hole in the eardrum. The memory of how I had saved her life by finding the aneurysm was never mentioned.

Eventually, she found a different doctor which prevented future annoyance. I guess I was supposed to be thankful she did not sue me. In truth, she did not suffer enough expense or endure enough pain to grab the attention of a lawyer.

The safest way to remove wax is with an operating microscope and suction.☼ In my experience, most family doctors have neither. It is your option to see a specialist for the removal of earwax. But in 40 years of irrigating ears, I had only one perforation with irrigation. There you have it.

Some information for making an informed decision about earwax removal.

The point of these two stories is that when a doctor helps you in an important way, let him/her know how much better you are. It will be appreciated. It will supply needed energy.

Hypothesis, Experimentation, Conclusion

In the scientific method, you need a hypothesis, a design of an experiment to test the validity of the hypothesis, and a written record of the results of the experiment. Only then do you draw a conclusion.

My son who is a physicist told me it's not science if you don't have a written record. In the well-run experiment, you need an independent variable, a dependent variable or outcome, and a control group.

But let's not make this too complicated

There are plenty of people in this life who develop theories and never take the time to test them. Most of us operate that way. As a doctor, I am from a tradition that goes back 1000s of years. For centuries, doctors based their practice on theories that no one ever got around to proving, I am sorry to say. Consider leeches. They were used for 2500 years.

In the medical field, it is better to use theories that have been tested and proven to work ☼ and that is always how I tried to practice.

But many times, you face a situation for which there is no proven method. You still need to help the patient. Decisions must be made without the benefit of definitive scientific evidence because the right studies have not yet been performed.

In the nonmedical arenas of life, I feel free to employ hypotheses that I never bothered to prove. That lack of experimentation would be considered sloppy to a bona fide scientist. If I figure out something and it seems to work, I do it. Skip the data collection and the experiments.

I don't think I'm different from most people in this regard. I mean lots of people seek to come up with different or unusual ideas or theories about how to best do this or that.

For example, I don't like stinky kitchen sponges and who does? I found out to my own satisfaction that if I microwave my sponges every few days and then let them dry out, they never get smelly. Hypothesis and conclusion only; no experiment, no controls, no written record.

For some treatments it is so obvious that they work they don't need proof with the scientific method. Like curing patients with leeches. Just kidding or am I? Surprisingly, we still use leeches. Plastic surgeons use them to treat some wound complications.

Someone said you don't need a university-based double-blind controlled study to prove it hurts to hit yourself on the head with a hammer. I cannot deny that.

But for treatment decisions about serious conditions that are not that obvious, look for guidelines based on good scientific studies.

Scientific Shaving

Ambrose Bierce (1842-1914) defined a story as "A narrative, commonly untrue." However, everything in the following story is true, except for the part about scientific shaving. I will admit that's just an untested hypothesis.

Rob Orr, the men's swimming coach at Princeton, retired in 2019 after 40 seasons, having won 330 dual meet victories and 23 Ivy League Championships. Shortly before he retired, he contacted me to ask, "What was this business I heard about "Scientific Shaving?"

In the sport of swimming, everyone accepts the idea that shaving the hair from a man's body just before a championship will significantly reduce drag and result in faster times. Has that been proven? No, not really.

Swimmers who shave down for a championship will nearly always swim faster. I can think of other reasons you would swim faster the day you shaved down. You have the advantage of entering the competition fully rested for these big meets. You are revved up psychologically. After shaving, you experience a sensory effect. The freshly shaved body feels different. You feel like a porpoise. You feel fast, amazingly fast. That gets you going psychologically.

At Princeton, the swimmers shaved every year for the big championships, in my day mainly for the Eastern intercollegiate meet. In 1969, when shaving down the night before that meet, I had an idea, a theory, a hypothesis.

It went like this: swimmers propel themselves with their pull using their hands. The better you grab the water, the more water you can throw behind you. That is what makes you go forward. Isn't it likely that some of the propulsion comes from the swimmer's forearms as well as from the hands? I knew I wanted a slippery, shaved body but did I really want slippery, shaved forearms? If I shaved them, wouldn't I lose some of that ability to grab the water as I pulled?

I was about to shave my forearms that night. I started with the tops and then I did the bottoms but I hesitated before shaving the sides. I decided I wanted my inner and outer forearm edge surfaces to grab that tiny extra amount of water during my pull.

I thought to myself, "Why not?" which was what we said before WTF was invented. So I did not finish the edges. That left a hairy one-inch strip on the sides of my forearms.

The next day on the pool deck, my teammates and my coach asked me about my odd-looking forearms. They could see a distinct stripe of hair-bearing skin from the base of my fifth finger to my elbow and a similar stripe on the thumb side of each forearm.

What could I say? I just said I was using "scientific shaving," which I explained was a method of increasing drag where it was needed.

How did I swim? Great! We all swam great. I recall doing my best splits on the relays.

That summer after my sophomore year, I did not swim competitively. I was aiming for medical school and I needed a job in the medical field.

That was something expected of medical school applicants. I had been lucky enough to land that morgue attendant job I described in an earlier chapter. At the office of the county coroner in Cincinnati, I assisted with one to three autopsies every day.

I did everything from tying on toe tags to removing the deceased's brains for the forensic pathologists.

While I was working in Cincinnati, my best friend, Art Deffaa, went to California to train with a coach named Pete Gambril. He was the premier swim coach in the United States at the time, and Art had the opportunity to work out with some of the best swimmers in the country. One of them was Rob Orr, mentioned at the top of this story, who was my age and a swimmer for USC, the University of Southern California.

In 1969, the Summer National Swimming Championships were held in Louisville Kentucky. I decided I would take the two-hour trip down the freeway from Cincinnati and see my friend Art swim in the big meet.

Art introduced me to some of the California swimmers he knew. I spent most of my time watching and studying the technique of America's best swimmers. I was a freestyler. Over my career I had learned a lot from watching great freestylers and I used what I had observed to try to improve my stroke mechanics. I reverently respected the abilities of America's top swimmers.

As I sat in the bleachers that afternoon, it grabbed my attention for sure when I saw the world's fastest freestyle swimmer approaching. He seemed to know exactly where he was going. He came up to me, reached out his arm to shake my hand, and asked if I were Bob Sinsheimer.

He told me that this guy from New Jersey, a guy with whom he worked out (my buddy Art) had told him about this new technique I had developed at Princeton, "Scientific Shaving." He had heard how I had taken my arms to the engineering department at Princeton and placed them in a wind tunnel where testing revealed the proper way to shave a freestyler's forearms.

What could I say to this young man, who I considered to be a "god" of my sport? I had to think fast.

How did I respond? I really don't remember exactly what I said. I know I didn't deny Art's story. I probably said, "It's nothing complicated, you just leave a hairy strip on the edges of your forearms so they can better grab the water."

I don't think I was a good enough liar to have fabricated elaborate details of my imagined scientific and engineering accomplishments. So I just went along with it.

It was an excellent prank both on me and on this great swimmer.

That was 1969. Fifty years later it's 2019 and Coach Orr has sent me an email: "Was it you that Art once told me went to the engineering wind tunnel to test shaving down?

Ah, the evil that men do lives on...

Getting back to the medical themes, my duty as an author requires me to point out that a lot of the theories that doctors and patients come to believe derive from old, dubious stories like this one. When somebody figures out a treatment and it works or seems to work, we talk about it. If the inventor has a grey head of hair and comes from a well-known medical school, the idea can become popular. One humorist said this is called "eminence-based medicine" as opposed to "evidence-based."

We call these success stories "anecdotal evidence." In medicine there is an expression about anecdotal evidence: "One case equals zero cases." In other words, they don't count. They don't prove a thing.

My story is true. Whether or not Scientific Shaving helps a swimmer with hairy forearms faster remains to be proven.

When your health is at stake and you're faced with a difficult decision, always check all the facts you can. Using anecdotal evidence is OK if the proposed treatment is not expensive and the condition is not urgent or serious. For example, if the doctor learned from another patient a trick to help relax and it worked with a few other patients, why not give it a try? But realize anecdotes are random. Sometimes doctors believe their own fictions but when it comes to big decisions, you don't need to believe them too.

☼ Look for evidence or what we call randomized-controlled studies.

Finally, a Treatment for Cold Sores

Type I Herpes Simplex virus is the cause of cold sores. I learned of this story because a medical student wrote about it in a letter to a medical journal years ago. It took place before doctors had antiviral medications which help cold sores a little bit by reducing by one or two days the usual seven to ten day duration of an outbreak.

A doctor once gave his patient a steroid injection for a joint problem. A week later, the patient reported that she had happened to be getting a cold sore on the day of the injection and usually those bother her for a week or more but this cold sore went away so quickly, she wondered if the steroid shot was responsible. (Yes, this is an example of an anecdote). The next time the doctor had a patient with a cold sore he administered a steroid injection just to see what would happen. The patient reported the cold sore promptly cleared up! He started treating cold sores with steroid injections. The word got out in the town and new patients came to him because they were bothered by recurrent cold sores too and their doctors could offer no effective treatment for them. He gave them steroid injections too.

The medical school assigned a student to the doctor for a month. The student asked the doctor why in the world he was giving steroid injections for herpes simplex infections.

In class, they had been taught that steroids could lead to more Herpes Simplex outbreaks.

The doctor explained how he had discovered this "treatment" from a patient's observation. The student threw down a challenge. The next three weeks, when patients came in for cold sore treatment, one would get steroids and the next one would get a saline injection, or salt water at the normal concentration found in the body which is harmless. The patients kept a log of their symptoms, carefully noting when the cold sore had healed.

If you have read this far in my book, you can guess the results. There was no difference in the two groups. The student wrote the letter to the journal to share the results. Herpes cold sores will go away on their own and people had just assumed the steroids were helping. The problem with this treatment: steroid injections can cause a number of adverse reactions that are predictable including raising the blood sugar and causing the bones to lose calcium. Anecdotal evidence is unreliable.

"Doctor, You are Not God"

Mary Shelley gave her novel <u>Frankenstein</u> a subtitle: "The Modern Prometheus".

In the Greek myth, the god Prometheus creates man from clay and then gives man fire, deeply angering the other gods. Man was not supposed to have fire.

Zeus has the rebellious Prometheus chained to a rock where eagles eat his liver every day but the liver grows back each night so the torture is eternal. The message: Fire is Godly stuff, if you distribute God's things to men you get punished. Or, Man should not be like God.

In 1816, Mary was 19 and she had just married her husband, the poet Percy Bysshe Shelley. To escape the terrible weather common in the British Isles, Englishmen would travel south. Percy and Mary went to Geneva, Switzerland with a group of Romance poets.

The poets' plan went awry when it rained in Geneva every day that month. Lord Byron suggested they each write a ghost story to pass the dark, rainy days. It was this bad weather that lead to the creation of Mary's inventive gothic novel about a monster brought to life from inanimate flesh.

Mary's story became the novel <u>Frankenstein</u>. Doctor Frankenstein creates a monster. The experiment works but is a disaster after the monster has a temper tantrum and murders Dr. Frankenstein's family. The moral: Frankenstein was punished for violating a critical law of God: only God gets to create life.

I think everyone who watched TV in the 1970s recalls the Chiffon margarine commercial. Mother Nature is fooled into trying Chiffon and identifies it as "My delicious butter," only to learn the spread is actually margarine. Mother Nature suddenly turns dark and utters the famous line, "It's not nice to fool Mother Nature!" which is followed by bolts of lightning.

Don't fool with Mother Nature! Don't do stuff that only God is supposed to do.

Whoops, that's kind of like the work doctors do every day: we alter the natural biology of people.

Doctors! Maybe we need to remember "M.D." means Medical Doctor not Medical Deity. Don't get so proud when you change the course of nature to help your patient. Don't let your patients think you're like a God.

It's safe to say that many subsequent stories in literature derived from the Frankenstein of Mary Shelley. In these stories, the fictional scientists who cross the line are nearly always punished for their hubris.

Nowadays, society has misgivings about automation. Where will people work if the robots take our jobs? In our stories, movies, and TV series, scientists create thinking, self-aware robots. It's natural to think that as robots get smarter they will become more like humans. In a number of science fiction works that I have enjoyed, the scientists mess up when they crossing the "only God creates life" line by building sentient robots.

Sentient means the robot can reason, it can feel emotion, and it can experience pain and pleasure. Most troublesome, the sentient robot has an instinct for self-preservation that eclipses the programmed command to serve mankind.

Consider the <u>Terminator</u> movies. Man develops Skynet, a super artificial intelligence system. Skynet becomes self-aware and figures out that man is the only thing that can harm it. Skynet launches a world war of robots against humans to eliminate mankind.

If you watched HBO's Westworld, which won nine primetime Emmy awards, you will know the robots strike back at the humans after they become sentient.

OK, we get it: only God is allowed to create life.

As doctors, we don't create life but we can extend it by managing disease. But it is God who both creates disease and cures disease.

Doctors might "discover" a cure but we usually don't create the cure.

Healing often means we just set up the right conditions so that God or nature can do the work. We make a vaccine, but the secret is we just inject something to trick the immune system into making antibodies to prepare us before we get exposed to the disease. The active stuff in the vaccine is derived from something in nature. The real work is done by our body. We prescribe an antibiotic but the secret is that most of the antibiotics we use were found in nature, starting with the mold that gave us penicillin.

We make a minor change to the body like removing the infected appendix but the body does all the cleanup work. We set a fracture but the body heals the bone.

When I was about 12, my father told me he had created me. What he said started me thinking. Later in medical school, I studied anatomy. I thought, if he had created me, he would have known how many bones were in my hand and how the muscles were attached and what chemicals my brain produces to make my hand move. You could say it's just semantics but a father just throws the switch. It isn't an act of creation. In a similar way of looking at it, doctors don't create healing or cures.

Doctors and nurses work within narrow confines of what is possible.

In the *practice* of medicine, we can only treat things for which a treatment has been discovered. In the *art* of medicine, we can go further. In our role as doctors and nurses we need to maintain a high degree of humility. We never deserve all the credit.

"He's One of the Best Doctors in Town, and If You Don't Believe Me, Just Ask Him."

Beware the "expert" who knows something no one else knows. Beware healers who confidently present ideas that make sense to them without offering a shred of bona fide test data. Beware practitioners who can offer no confirmation that acceptable scientific standards have been achieved to prove that their idea or their treatment works.

These promoters often go by what makes sense to them. They deny the process of medical science. The work of real medical scientists is often denounced or even vilified as part of a conspiracy to defeat progress, to maintain the *status quo, or* to protect profits.

You may even discover a self-impressed charlatan who works for his cause at no profit for himself. He/she sincerely feels that his/her ideas are Nobel prize-worthy. Maybe they are not in it for the money. When a kook spreads his medical treatment ideas purely out of a love of mankind, that does not mean those ideas are trustworthy. Recall the expression: "The road to hell is paved with good intentions."

We still need to see their new evidence when the current practice with which they disagree was based on evidence. Or we need to see the opinion of experts who are qualified to evaluate the evidence and then provide an opinion on whether the treatment makes sense.

Modern medicine is not purely the result of science. For many conditions, we don't have irrefutable proof that traditional care works.

For some treatments, a double-blind study cannot be done. We can't devise a new vaccine for a fatal illness, give it to half the test subjects, give a placebo to the other half, and then deliberately infect the entire group and dutifully wait to record who lives and who dies.

Yet we are under great pressure to do SOMETHING for the patient. Consider what Voltaire (1694-1778) wrote: "L'art de la medecine consiste a distraire le patient pendant que la nature le guerit."

"The art of medicine consists of distracting (or amusing) the patient while nature cures the disease."

It's easier to detect bias in the person who has something to gain from you financially if you accept the treatment they offer. That bias is explicit.

But intellectual hubris is a type of implicit bias. It is ingrained. The seller sincerely believes he is helping his fellow man and the most perceptive patient will detect no sign of insincerely or falsehood.

Dr. Frankenstein's fatal flaw was pride. In the same way, consider the bias of pride in the "experts" whose cures were invented in someone's head, rather than developed and proven with the scientific method.

Remember, the best scientists constantly doubt their work and look for what's wrong. Charles Darwin's theory was arguably the most important scientific achievement of the 19th century. He came up with his ideas before we understood DNA. Yet Darwin had serious self-doubts after developing his concept of evolution.

In my experience, the best doctors are *modest*. I am wary of the pride of the overconfident doctor.

I remember some doctors who had huge, financially successful practices. Many patients were mesmerized by the quality of their office furnishings or the cut of the doctor's suit. Some of these doctors were not respected by their peers. Patients who had heard the buzz might ask me, what did I think about Dr. So and So, one of those marvelous doctors who were marvelously high-income and marvelously self-promoting. I would sometimes wink and say, "He's one of the best doctors in town, and if you don't believe me, just ask him."

So when someone brings out a novel idea about health, take it with a mixture of interest and skepticism. Consider the explicit and implicit bias. Look for well-run studies or guidelines from respected sources.

Keeping Track of your Systolic Blood Pressure

Always look for ways to make one thing easier. When you keep track of your blood pressure over the age of 50, you mainly need to pay attention to the top number or systolic. Systolic is the one that matters as we age. ☼

What is systolic? Imagine we have a little tiny needle that goes into an artery and is connected to a pressure meter. It gives a continuous reading of the pressure and makes a graph. As the heart beats the pressure goes up. Then it starts to slowly fall until the heart beats again when it goes up again. The resulting graph would be a sawtooth pattern of ups and downs, like hills and valleys. The top of the hill is the systolic pressure, and the bottom is the diastolic.

Yes, for years we told you that the diastolic was more important. True, the heart spends more time near the diastolic pressure than the systolic, so the lower diastolic figure should matter more. In our minds, the diastolic matters more. But statistics show the risk of heart attack and stroke correlates with the systolic reading. ☼ Just look at the stroke risk calculators or the heart attack risk calculators or the combined stroke and heart attack risk calculators. They don't ask about your diastolic, just the systolic.

Generally over the age of 50, if the systolic is good the diastolic will be good.

So if a patient said, "My blood pressure averages 121 over something okay," I knew what I needed to know.

I have observed when patients respond to that inner, compulsive desire to remember both numbers, they may get the systolic wrong.

But you're not going to memorize your readings. You are going to write them down because as a reader of this book, you are a sensible person.

By the way, if you keep track of your blood pressure, and that's an excellent idea, don't bring the doctor all 80 readings since the last visit.

The doctor might be an arithmetic whiz, but even Einstein types cannot look at that string of numbers and figure out the average in an eyeblink. If the numbers vary a lot, work out the average for your doctor. If they are fairly consistent` you can simply tell the doctor something like: "I took 25 readings and all but three were under 125 systolic."

Remember: do record the date, the systolic and diastolic, and which arm.

If one arm is always higher, that's the accurate one. When one arm is always lower there may be a narrowing in an artery on the low side.☼ That arm is not telling you the systolic BP your brain and heart are feeling.

Once in a while, you need to compare both your arms. I recall in my early years of practice a lady came in as a new patient with a complaint of lightheadedness. She said at her former doctor's office, whenever the nurse tried to check her blood pressure, she couldn't hear it. The doctor would check it and say, "I don't know what the problem is, I hear it fine." A lightbulb turned on in my brain. I checked the pulse in both arms. One was normal but the other was very faint. It turned out that the nurse always liked to check BP on the left arm but the doctor always liked to check it on the right arm. She had a condition called "Subclavian Steal Syndrome." The artery that went to the one arm was blocked so the body fed the arm by stealing blood from the brain via the vertebral artery to the subclavian artery just past the blockage. That was why she was lightheaded. The problem was resolved after surgical repair of the arteries.

Write them down: The idea that you can keep track of your blood pressure readings in your head is delusional.

Swimming Forever

I saw this on a button for sale at a swimming meet.

"If the doctor ever tells me I only have one day to live I want to go to a swim meet. They go on forever."

USA Swimming has meets that go on for three days. I once competed in a Master's World Swimming Championship meet in Munich, Germany, which took six days. They held three events per day, starting at 7 a.m. and finishing around 11 p.m. Imagine a baseball game that lasted six days!

When I was swimming as a kid 60 years ago in New Jersey, it was different. The New Jersey branch of the Amateur Athletic Union, or AAU, which was in charge before USA Swimming, held meets with only ten events. There was one race for each age group, boys and girls 10 and under, 11&12, 13&14, 15–18, and then open or senior championship events. For each race, the meet started with the preliminary heats followed by a ten-minute break and then they held ten more races at the end. These were the finals. They were very exciting because the medals were decided in the finals. Four-lane pool, three medals. Lots of motivation there.

Today I only see finals in the State High School Championships, National and other championships and big international meets such as the Olympics.

Those ten event New Jersey meets in the '60s were fun. They only lasted three hours or so. You only had one race to swim so when you swam your race, you competed against everyone in the state who came to the meet in your age group. They announced the swimmers in each lane before running each heat. The finals were very exciting, the climax of the evening.

On the way home, we stopped for hamburgers and milkshakes at Howard Johnson's. There was only one Mcdonald's in the entire state of New Jersey back then.

In today's swim meets they have ten events in each age group and the meets start Friday night, and then continue all day Saturday and Sunday. It's exhausting. They usually have "timed finals," which means no finals. The final ranking is based on the time in the heats. The swimmers in the fastest heat might think they are battling for the gold medal, but someone from an earlier heat wins due to having a faster time. Because there are so many events in your age group, you cannot swim in every event.

But in New Jersey back then, everyone swam every event because they only had one event for your age group. You might wonder if it was worth traveling to a meet for one event, but New Jersey is a small state and most of the population is near New York City.

In those days a swim meet did not seem like forever. And as I get older, swimming forever seems like a good idea.

If you keep on swimming, you certainly feel like you're going to live longer. You are energized. But don't swim too

198

hard. When you get older, just go fast enough to keep it a little interesting.

When I work out I typically do 100 yards, rest for 60 plus seconds then go again. As the years pass, my swimming times are definitely slower, but those one-minute rests seem quicker.

When I was 46, I went to my first Master's National Championship, the first National competition I'd been to since I was in college.

I entered the natatorium to look around. I couldn't believe how many swimmers of all ages were warming up in the huge pool at the University of Michigan.

Suddenly I noticed an ancient-looking man walking towards me. When he was five feet away he reached out his hand.

"Sinsheimer, how are you?"

It was Mickey Vogt, my freshman swim coach who had retired in 1968. This was 1996, 28 years later and he was 91. There were five swimmers in his age group, 90–94, and naturally, he won a medal in every race.

Mickey told me that if you swim every other day for the rest of your life, one day people will say, "He died the day he went swimming." or "He died the day after he went swimming." I said, "And if you quit swimming, they'll say, 'You know he used to swim every other day but then he quit and died.' "

Mickey reached the far end of the pool at age 97. I don't know if he had continued to swim every other day. I think so because in the obituary they pointed out that he had worked out two days before he passed. Close enough.

I hope I can swim forever. Every year I get a little slower. I think if I keep getting slower and slower every year, eventually, I'll be swimming backward.

Wilby

When I was ten at my very first AAU swim meet, I thought I heard them announce this guy named Wilby who was swimming in the next heat. I kept hearing his name over and over that day.

I would hear something like, "Heat three, lane one: Johnny Smith, lane two: Harry Jones, lane three Pete Peterson, lane four: Wilby Oben. But when my 10-year-old eyes looked for Wilby in lane four, I would just see an open lane.

Eventually I got it: Lane four: Will be open.

Perspectives on Death

"I am not afraid of death, I just don't want to be there when it happens." Woody Allen.

"I did not attend his funeral, but I sent a nice letter saying I approved of it." Mark Twain.

I like this story about the minister, the priest, and the rabbi who were at the funeral of a friend:

The minister said, "I hope when I'm lying in my casket, people will say 'He was a good man and was devout in his dedication to Jesus.' "

The priest said, "I hope when I'm there, people will say 'He led his parish in faith and helped them to become better people' ".

And the rabbi said, "When I'm lying there I hope someone says, 'Look, I just saw his leg move!' "

Don't Tell Dad He's Dying

I remember a rather sick, elderly man whose family approached me before I entered the exam room and firmly commanded me not to tell him that he was dying of his advanced heart failure. They thought withholding the truth would be the kindest approach.

I felt conflicted. Didn't my patient deserve to know the truth? But to disclose that he was dying might cause psychological reverberations that the family would have to deal with, not me. I concluded that telling him was a bad idea and so was not telling him. I decided to tiptoe around the subject.

At an appropriate time during the visit, after he had described all the symptoms that were troubling him and how his symptoms had failed to improve after cardiology consultations and recommended treatments, I simply asked him if he were worried about dying.

He said something like this: "Oh no, I know I'm dying, I think it's my time. Just don't tell my family, it will get them worried."

Dilator For Blood Pressure

This is a true story. One day a patient I knew well came in for a routine hypertension follow-up visit.

He said, "Doctor, can you put me on a dilator."

Indeed, we have a class of drugs called vasodilators which lower blood pressure by dilating or opening up the arteries. Sometimes they work so well that the patient winds up with some swelling in the legs because the medication augments the arterial flow down to the legs without improving the venous return up the lower extremities back to the heart.

After he asked me the question, I thought to myself, "He's not taking a vasodilator now. Why did he ask for that particular class of drug?

I wasn't sure we were communicating so I said, "A dilator? Patients don't usually use that terminology. What do you have in mind?"

"I don't know," he said. "I just heard there are blood pressure drugs called dilators and I thought I should be on one."

"Why?"

"Because you die later, isn't that the idea?

Lead Time Bias in the Evaluation of Cancer Success, Part 1 (Principles)

Lead time must be understood when discussing cancer "survival times." This is "lead" rhymes with deed not lead rhymes with dead. Whether you really understand "survival time" is not something the people "behind the curtain" worry about much. Unfortunately focusing on the "five-year survival" can fool people.

"FIVE YEAR SURVIVAL" in the NCI (National Cancer Institute) dictionary of cancer terms: "The percentage of people in a study or treatment group who are alive five years after they were diagnosed with or started treatment for a disease, such as cancer."

Former New York City Mayor Rudolph Giuliani was discussed in an editorial in the British Medical Journal in February 2013. When Mr. Giuliani was running for president in 2007, he trumpeted the superiority of American Medicine because as an American, his chance of a five-year survival after receiving treatment for his prostate cancer was 82% compared with only 44% in England. Giuliani used this statistic to try to prove that socialized medicine in Britain is inferior. As the editorial points out, "Yet despite this impressive difference in the five-year survival rate, the mortality rate is about the same in the United States and the United Kingdom."

Gigerenzer, Gerd and Wegwarth, Odette. "Five year survival rates can mislead" British Medical Journal February 2, 2013 volume 364 page 24

What can explain these stats?

Survival time is the difference between when the cancer starts and when the patient dies from it. Exactly when should we start the clock when measuring survival time? The survival time clock that should matter would start when the cancer arose, the date the cancer cells first appeared in the patient.

That's logical but it is impractical. We never know that actual date the cancer first appeared. The first cell to turn cancerous could have been there for a decade before it became detectable with a test. So, let's say we should start the timer at the earliest time the cancer could have shown up on any existing diagnostic test.

The cancer principle nearly everyone believes in, as firmly as the belief that the sun rises in the east and rivers flow downstream, is that when we make the cancer diagnosis early and treatment is effective, the survival time will be longer. But survival time from the earliest possible date of detection is not something we can usually determine either. What we can use as the start time can be found in the patient's medical record. The clock was started when the cancer was discovered.

There is no dispute about the survival end time, death of the patient. There's a public record on that.

But the difference between the cancer's actual start date and the one we use, the date of diagnosis, can be years.

So if a patient's cancer could have been detected in 2005 but we found it in 2010 and the patient died in 2015, was that a ten-year survival or a five-year survival?

The overestimation of the extra years of survival due to earlier screening is called the lead time bias. Even if you decide not to treat the cancer, finding it early with screening adds to the "survival time." If the screening helps you find it two years earlier, the survival time automatically goes up by two years. That makes people biased in favor of screening tests.

The lead time factor is not considered in cancer statistics that focus on "Five Year Survival." In a single sentence: if you found the tumor earlier by cancer screening, the early survival years are extended and the cancer business looks better. It does not matter if the date of death was not extended.

It blows my mind that patients don't know about lead time bias.

I just saw a website for a blood test that claims to find cancer early. They advertise "In fact, when cancers are diagnosed early before they have the chance to spread, the overall five-year survival rate is four times higher than when diagnosed in later stages." That's amazing. Even without understanding the contribution of lead-time bias, are we not supposed to be smart enough to figure out that if the five-year survival were 30% and with their test it is four times that, we have 4x30=120 or 120% five-year survival. How can you have a 120% five-year survival rate? That would mean for every 100 patients found with their test, 120 of those live five years. Where did they get the extra 20 people? Once a retired math teacher told me that 5 out of four people don't understand fractions. That's an absurd claim. Early cancer detection by new tumor markers are bound to work just like the old tumor markers: a few are useful, many cause false alarms that require extenstive testing none-the-less, and most just cause unhappiness without truly extending the life of cancer patients..

Lead-Time Bias Part 2: the Story of Pete and Re-Pete

If you get what I'm saying about lead-time bias, you can skip this chapter. I'm going to make the same point but with a story.

I like to give the example of two twin brothers we will call Pete and Re-Pete. Due to identical genes they were identical in appearance but not only that. By a freak of nature, they were identical in all life events from birth. What happened medically to one always happened to the other one and nearly at the same time. If one fell down the steps and broke his arm the other did the same during the same week. If one developed an ulcer, the other developed an ulcer. These co-occurrences happened even if they were living apart. They would have lived their lives in parallel, even if they had been separated at birth and adopted into different families.

I would point out that if a cancer started growing in one, so it did in the other one and at the same time.

This story sounds like science fiction. Pete and Re-Pete had lives too peculiarly coincidental to be real. But they represent a good case for illustrative purposes because the brothers represent statistical averages.

What I mean is if you take a few million people in one group and the same number of similar people in another, the number of cancers, and the average age of cancer onset will average the same. The number falling down stairs during a particular month will be equal too, as long as the two groups are very large. The number who play baseball and the number who are high school class valedictorians would be equal, except for that high school in whichever state it was that had so much grade inflation that half the class had a 4.0 average and were all named valedictorians.

So considering these two remarkable twins, Peter and Re-Pete, it turns out that after they grew up they went to different family doctors. Both would go in yearly for a wellness exam where screening tests were performed or not. Peter's doctor was conventional, meaning that he performed all the tests that were recommended by experts and that was all.

But Re-Pete's doctor thought that he would go the extra mile for his patients. He did a lot more testing than experts recommended. Re-Pete's doctor periodically ordered CT scans of the chest and abdomen and over the years they found a lot of things that Peter's doctor never discovered! CT scans are good at that!

Nowadays this doctor would probably order one of those $949 blood DNA tests not covered by insurance that claim to discover many types of cancer for which we do not currently screen.

Re-Pete had quite a number of false alarms over the years that resulted in additional testing and expense. Sometimes the pursuit of these findings resulted in suffering pain from biopsies performed with long needles stuck into some difficult-to-reach internal organs. One time the needle nicked an artery during a biopsy and Re-Pete had to undergo surgery to stop the bleeding. Re-Pete also suffered a loss of time from work and not a little expense from all the extra testing.

When Re-Pete turned 45 his doctor ordered a CT of the abdomen as a screening test. It showed a very early cancer of the pancreas. Re-Pete's doctor considered this discovery to be a triumph of early detection! Re-Pete was treated for this cancer in the usual way with radiation therapy and chemotherapy. But poor Re-Pete was never the same after this; the treatment caused some side effects that affected him for the rest of his life. He was happy to be alive yet his happiness was blunted because he was haunted by thoughts that he had suffered a very serious type of cancer that could come back at any time.

Unfortunately, cancer of the pancreas is a very difficult and tricky opponent. It tends to surreptitiously spread microscopically around the body before it can be seen on a CT scan or other test. That happens more often than we know because if the cancer cells grow slowly and the patient is older, we never find out.

Although the doctors declared that Re-Pete had been cured, that all the cancer was removed, indeed he had tiny, slowly growing metastatic nests of cancer all over his body. Nine and a half years later, a return of the cancer was discovered in the liver. This particular tumor did not respond to radiation or chemotherapy. That's not uncommon with pancreatic cancer. Re-Pete was very sick for six months and passed away on his birthday at age 55.

At his funeral, his son publicly thanked the doctor for helping his father survive pancreatic cancer for a remarkable ten years thanks to early screening and detection! We would record that Re-Pete had a ten-year survival from pancreatic cancer.

Now Re-Pete's brother Pete also went to a family doctor. Pete's doctor did not do these extra CT scans. Pete's doctor played by the rules and those screening scans were not recommended by experts. Because he was medically identical to his brother, at age 45 Pete also had developed a cancer of the pancreas large enough to be discovered by a CT scan, but it did not cause symptoms so it wasn't discovered. And he also had very tiny metastatic cells in his liver and other places that were too small to be discovered. These cancerous cells divided and multiplied like his brother's tumors.

Pete did not get the chemotherapy treatment or the radiation that his brother did. Let's point out that Re-Pete's tumors did shrink a little with therapy but sometimes it's like dandelions on the lawn. If you pull them and leave some of the root behind, they're all back in a few weeks.

Pete escaped the worry of knowing he had cancer. He escaped being sick from the chemotherapy and radiation.

When Pete was 54, he started feeling sick. At first, he seemed to be responding to an ulcer medication, but it was soon obvious that something was seriously wrong. A CT scan showed pancreatic cancer with spread to the liver. For one year Pete endured powerful chemotherapy and radiation therapy and suffered the sad knowledge that he had a serious, life-threatening malignancy. After the treatments did not make the cancer shrink much, the doctors declared that this tumor type was resistant to therapy.

On his birthday at age 55, Pete died, the same day as his brother. We would record that Pete had a one-year survival from pancreatic cancer.

At his funeral, there were mumblings that maybe Pete's doctor should be sued for failure to make an earlier diagnosis. Look how well his brother did, a ten-year cancer survivor!

So what do we have here?

Re-Pete was treated early, endured ten years of side effects from his treatment and ten years of stress knowing he had a serious life-threatening cancer plus considerable expense. Re-Pete survived ten years.

Pete was treated late and survived for only one year. Before that he had nine years of blissful ignorance. Re-Pete's doctor was praised. Pete's doctor might have been sued. Both brothers died the same day on their 55th birthday.

Early detection resulted in ten times longer survival for Re-Pete. Clearly ten years of survival is better than one year of survival, right? Right? No...I'm being ironic.

Early detection: In this example it doesn't look like such a good deal.

A Riddle Wrapped in a Mystery Inside an Enigma.

Winston Churchill said that; he was talking about the Soviet Union. We could say the same about the screening for and treating cancer. Evaluation how we screen for and treat cancer is complex.

Someone said, "The secret of a long life is to develop a chronic illness and keep it for a long time."

My story of Pete and Re-Pete is just one possible scenario for pancreatic cancer. It is based on the notion that the tumor was resistant to treatment. Sometimes that is the case, but sometimes early therapy is remarkably effective.

If you want to know which cancers are the best ones to screen for, the very difficult and mathematically challenging research and analysis has already been done for you. Look at the recommendations of the United State Preventive Services Task Force or USPSTF. They've worked out the statistics. Screening is a good idea for only a few types of cancer.

To explain why some cancers don't lend themselves to smart screening, let's describe the perfect cancer screening test.

First, there should be a long "window of opportunity," a period when the cancer is present but early enough to cause nearly no symptoms and yet large enough to be detected on the screening test.

If that window only lasted only a month, then screening is impractical. You might as well wait a month for symptoms to develop symptoms and then test when the patient comes in.

Second, treatment success must be much higher when the cancer is found earlier because of testing during that screening window. The ideal cancer is found before there is any visible spread and before there is any microscopic spread. Finding cancer after it's spread is like closing the barn door after the horse got out.

Third, a slow-growing cancer that does not respond to treatment does not need to be found early by screening.

Fourth, the test must be affordable to society and

Fifth, not so unpleasant that people refuse it.

For one cancer early detection not only can cure but it works on all patients. I am referring to cancer of the uterine cervix. The Pap smear is really great! It takes over a decade for the positive Pap to evolve into incurable invasive cancer of the cervix. That's a huge window.

Second criterion: treatment success is high when it is found early. Nearly 100% for the Pap smear.

Third: treatment is effective. Fourth: the Pap test is affordable. Fifth: paps are not painful (if done right).

If every woman of the proper ages per the guidelines gets a Pap smear every 5 years, there will be nearly zero deaths from cancer of the cervix.

For some other cancers, it might only be 50% of those detected and treated early who actually do better from early detection. Or 10% benefiting. Or 1%.

We cannot judge our success in treatment with five-year survival stats. We need to look at the overall death rate from that cancer in the US population. If the five-year stats get better but the cancer deaths from that type of cancer do not fall, we need to do some looking behind the curtain.

The point of this discussion is that part of the gain produced by early detection with cancer screening is an illusion. I think patients deserve to know it can happen both ways. Early detection can be wonderful, but early detection can also be a wasteful illusion. Sorry, it's not black and white.

There's an ironic side to this conundrum. When looking at cancer success stories, the best cancers to have are the ones that are labeled as cases of "overdiagnosis." They are the cancers that did not need to be found at all, because they grow so slowly that the patient died of something else before the cancer became active enough to cause symptoms.

When each and every one of these "overdiagnosis" or "not needing to be found" cancers, are treated, everybody labels them as a success story! The patient was treated and did not die from the cancer! For our profession to accept credit for these saves is fraudulent.☼

A lot of slower-growing tumors in the elderly fit into this category. ☼ It's good that is some cases, when you slow down due to age, your cancer's growth rate slows down too.

Of course, treating those overdiagnosed cancers won't help the overall US death rate from that cancer.

Only research can distinguish the ratio of real successes from the imagined ones.

Preventative medicine experts struggle to know which cancers are best to find early and which are not. Which need to be treated early?

The reason for you to know about lead-time bias is to understand why screening is only recommended for a few cancers. We don't screen for leukemia, for esophageal cancer, for bone cancer, for liver cancer, for pancreatic cancer etc.

Aggressive cancer screening, and by that I mean getting more testing than recommended by screening experts, is *nearly always going to be a bad idea.* Now you know why. Now it should not sound so bizarre to hear that a certain cancer did not need to be found early or that another cancer did not need to be treated.

I think we need to shift our energy from screening to prevention. We need to avoid chemicals that cause cancer (carcinogens). Keeping our weight down, avoiding moderate or heavy drinking, avoiding sunburn, and many other measures have a good effect on your effort to avoid cancer.

A Guy Goes Into a Bar

I heard that whether fiction or non-fiction, every book has "dry" sections. I hope the last three chapters about lead time bias were interesting and you learned something that you never knew. In case you were just bored to tears, here's a story that also has to do with interpreting numbers. It's a drinking joke so it can't be "dry."

A guy goes to a bar and orders three beers. The bartender thinks he was ordering for himself and a few friends but he just sits down and proceeds to drink all three himself. The bartender says to him, "You know, it might be better to order one at a time. The third beer could go flat on you."

The customer says, "Let me explain. I have two brothers. We always used to drink together. But now Mikey is in Australia and Petey is in England. So when we go to a bar, we always order three. I drink this one, that's for Petey. I drink that one, that's for Mikey. I drink the third one, that's for me.

The bartender says, "That's a nice way to remember the good times with your brothers."

The guy becomes a regular at the bar. He always orders three beers. Sometimes six. Or nine. Or twelve.

One day he comes in and only orders two beers.

His friend the bartender comes over and says, "I don't want to pry, but is your family OK?"

The customer looks confused for a moment. Then he brightens up. He says, "Oh, no...my brothers are fine. It's me! I quit drinking."

The Value of Dogs and Other Pets

Did you hear about the agnostic who was also dyslexic and a chronic insomniac? No?

He was up all night wondering if there really was a dog.

Dogs have a high place in many homes. Maybe not as elevated as God the Father, but certainly the dog is a full-fledged member of the family who outranks the husband of the dog owner.

Ambrose Bierce (1842-1914) referred to the dog as an incarnation, which means when God is transformed into the flesh. He wrote in his Devil's Dictionary that a dog is: "A kind of additional or subsidiary Deity designed to catch the overflow and surplus of the world's worship. This Divine Being in some of his smaller and silkier incarnations takes, in the affection of Woman, the place to which there is no human male aspirant."

Here is something your doctor might not have time to mention: Pets are important to our health, especially our mental health and possibly even our immune systems.

Groucho Marx said, "Outside of a dog, a book is man's best friend, but inside of a dog it's too dark to read."

I always tried to learn what patients did in life, and whenever I found out a patient raised dogs professionally, I would say, "Do you know you practice in the mental health field?"

And the patient would usually answer, "Yes, I know."

My advice to patients was to get a pet. A pet helps you get more exercise. A pet helps you meet people in the park.

214

A pet provides someone to take care of, someone to talk to. A pet offers a companion who never has a word of criticism.

Why do dogs matter to their owners? In a word, loyalty.

For tourists to Tokyo, a popular destination is the Shibuya train station. They will find a bronze statue of a dog outside. It is an Akita.

I learned that Akitas have been bred in Japan for 4000 years. The Akita is known to be dignified, courageous, and extremely loyal to its family and master.

I saw the 2009 movie <u>Hachi, a Dog's Tale</u>. It is a wonderful dog-lover's film based on a true story about an Akita named Hachiko, who every day walked with his master, a college professor, from home to the train station from which the professor commuted. At the end of the day, the dog was waiting for the master's train at the station. One day the professor suddenly died in front of his class. From 1925 to 1935 Hachiko waited for his master to return to that train station day and night, winter and summer. People noticed him and fed him. When he finally died of natural causes, folks erected a bronze statue to honor the dog and commemorate his incredible loyalty.

<u>A Dog's Tale</u> was a remake of an earlier Japanese film. It stared Richard Gere, Joan Allen, Sarah Roemer, Jason Alexander, and Erick Avari. If you don't recognize all the names, you will recognize the actors. The director was Lasse Hallstrom, who did Gilbert Grape, Chocolat, and The Cider House Rules.

For me, this story recalls Argos, a dog from the Odyssey, the epic poem composed 2800 years ago by Homer. Not many people remember the story of Argos, which is a shame.

Argos was Odysseus' dog. When Odysseus left Ithaca for the Trojan War, Argos was a young dog, having just been trained by his master.

As we learned in school, Odysseus spent ten years fighting in Troy, followed by ten more years wandering the Aegean Sea, enduring many dangerous adventures. He was the only Greek from Ithaca to return home. After those twenty years, his people assumed he had died.

A gang of suitors, taking advantage of the Greek tradition of unquestioning hospitality, occupied his house, believing that one of them would eventually be chosen as a new husband for the Queen, Penelope, who Odysseus had left behind. She remained unwaveringly faithful to Odysseus and resisted the suitors. Nevertheless, the suitors would not leave and held a continuous party at Penelope's expense.

Odysseus arrived on the shore of Ithaca, his journey over but one challenge remaining. The plan was for him to surreptitiously enter his home and attack the suitors. The goddess Athena physically transformed him into the shape of an elderly beggar. Only Telemachos, his son, now a 20-year-old, was told of his arrival.

As Odysseus approached his home, he found his dog Argos lying next to a pile of cow manure. Now over twenty years old, Argos was covered with fleas, ignoring everything and being ignored by all. Argos was once known for his speed and strength and his superior tracking skills. At this point in life, he spent the day lying down as if half-dead and moved slowly with the arthritis of old age.

Despite Odysseus' physical disguise, Argos recognized him at once. He had just enough strength to wag his tail and lift his head. But he was too weak to get up to greet his master. Even petting Argos might have betrayed his identity, so Odysseus was unable to acknowledge his beloved dog. He silently passed by Argos with a single tear and entered his home. Homer tells us that Argos' heart was broken, but his steadfast mission to see his master one more time had been completed, and he passed into the darkness of death.

—adapted from Homer, <u>Odyssey</u>, Book 17, lines 290-327

You Don't Need To Live Alone

Ambrose Bierce, who I have enjoyed reading since I was 16, wrote that to be alone was to be in good company.

I get that. It's OK to be alone for a few hours. It's peaceful. You can get stuff done when you're not interrupted. But day after day, I think it's better to have companionship.

The origin of the word *companion* is interesting. It derives from the Latin *com* meaning "with" and *panis* meaning "bread." A companion is someone with whom you share bread. Or your home. Or your time.

If you have no people with whom to share your life, get a dog if you can. If you're getting older, make it smaller to medium-sized.

If you live without other humans, make sure you have a backup person to watch your critter should you need to go to the hospital. I have had patients who refused to be hospitalized because they had nobody to watch their dog.

People love to help their neighbors, so if you live alone, don't be afraid to ask a neighbor to be the designated dog-sitter, should you be hospitalized suddenly.

I have read a dog can help the immune system. I don't know if the evidence for that theory is strong but this is an example of an harmless hypothesis. It's not important if someone later proves dogs don't help our immune systems. You are not going to sign up for "dog treatment" instead of critical medication that has shown to be effective.

Some experts think that exposure to animal dander stimulates the immune system of babies so they are better at resisting germs. A study from 2004 found that the secretion of immunoglobulin A (IgA) was increased in college students who petted dogs compared with those who petted a stuffed animal or nothing.

IgA levels are not obvious. Maybe those IgA increases were too small to matter. So the immune boosting hypothesis is not proven. But there are obvious benefits like the exercise from walking the dog. And the biggest benefit is living with a companion who will never criticize you and will always love you as long as you praise it and feed it. By the way, that's not a bad way to get along with people either.

What about other animals for pets?

I think to feel like your pet is your companion, you need one that can look you in the eye. Cats make the grade. I don't personally relate to a reptile or fish that has one eye on either side of its head looking out in different directions. But even any living pet may serve the purpose. People enjoy snakes, iguanas, fish and turtles.

Hilaire Belloc (1870-1953), an Anglo French satirist, wrote about having a pet amphibian in his poem, "The Frog." This is an impressively silly poem.

> Be kind and tender to the Frog,
>   And do not call him names,
> As 'Slimy skin,' or 'Polly-wog,'
>   Or likewise 'Ugly James,'
> Or 'Gape-a-grin,' or 'Toad-gone-wrong,'
>   Or 'Billy Bandy-knees':
> The Frog is justly sensitive
>   To epithets like these.
>
> No animal will more repay
>   A treatment kind and fair;
> At least so lonely people say
> Who keep a frog (and, by the way,
>   They are extremely rare).

READY, FIRE, AIM/ Evaluating For Reasonable Possibilities

The rule should be ready, aim, fire! Sometimes we see doctors, the really speedy doctors, do this: ready, FIRE.

They skip the aiming part.

Years ago, I heard the Chief of Medicine at our hospital refer to one of the busiest yet intellectually weak doctors on our staff: "His differential diagnosis is one horse, no zebras." When you are napping under a tree in the Midwest and you hear hoofbeats, a horse is what you expect to see. Zebras would not be expected. But in medicine, zebras show up all the time.

The patient must be prepared for this doctor-type. ☼ If your doctor seems to be going with the most likely possibility without considering other ones, you need to say something like this: "Doctor, are there any other possible causes of these symptoms that are reasonably possible even if not probable for which a delay would be disastrous?" Notice those two concepts "Possible" and "Probable." They sound like synonyms; they are not. In regards to the rain forecast, probable means the chance of rain is over 50%. Possible means any chance of rain, even 1%.

Over twenty years ago, I had a patient who was habituated to pain meds. She never had a problem with drugs before doctors started giving her narcotics for chronic pain but then the pain never went away and she couldn't stop the prescription pain pills. She took a lot when I met her but it was the same amount every day. Such a patient is not classified as a person with an addiction. ☼

To some doctors, she might have been just a lady who wanted pills. But I recognized she was functioning in life, holding a full-time job, and caring for her two children. So I continued her pain medication at the same level which she never exceeded. I knew that because we counted the days

219

between refills. Her urine tests confirmed she was taking as prescribed.

One day she went to the ED (emergency department) with abdominal pain and vomiting and subsequently was sent to a surgeon.

She related to me a day later that the surgeon told her that there was nothing wrong with her and to quit wasting his time.

This surgeon had experience with drug-seeking patients. So does every doctor. He thought that the greatest probability was that she only wanted pain medication. He forgot the reasonable possibilities of the case.

I was her family doctor, so she came to see me the next day. I listened. You say something to the patient like: "Tell me what's going on and everything that's important." You take notes while the patient talks. You clarify what's not clear, hopefully without interrupting the patient's train of thought.

One of the many things she told me about her condition was that the vomit smelled awful. That was my clue. I told her not to worry about the surgeon's opinion. I tested her further. We found her stomach had developed an ulcer which had penetrated the colon to forming an improper connection known as a gastro-colic fistula.

That meant she had an abnormal opening between the stomach and the stool in her colon. That was why the vomit smelled so bad. It smelled of stool. I sent her to the hospital under the care of a different surgeon. She had extensive major surgery and suffered a lengthy but successful recovery.

Let me assure you, the "ready-fire" surgeon whose "time was being wasted" was not involved in her care.

We sometimes see another type of doctor: ready, aim, aim, aim, aim, aim, fix something caused by the testing, and then fire (eventually, maybe).

If the doctor recommends extensive or overly aggressive (possibly harmful) testing or treatment, can you say this to your doctor: "Doctor, can we just give this some time? Would it be OK to see if the symptoms go away? If we did that are there any 'reasonable' possibilities that we might miss, something that would be really bad not to catch earlier?"

The key concept of possible here is reasonableness. In a lot of situations, the one chance in a million is not a reasonable possibility. There is always one chance in a million of something. Like being hit by a meteor. Like finding a real diamond ring in a Cracker Jack box. Like finding a gold nugget in an abandoned gold mine.

You wouldn't do financial planning based on a belief that you are going to win the lottery. Yes, somebody wins the lottery for sure. But believing you are going to win the lottery is not a reasonable expectation. It's usually delusional. I think most people who buy a lottery ticket think that way, if for only a moment.

How does the low probability of having the winning lottery ticket translate to medical choices? One chance in ten is certainly reasonable. One chance in 100 might be reasonable. For example the "Do-I-call the ambulance-for-chest-pain-because-it-might-be-a-heart-attack" decision: If there were one chance in 100 that the symptom represented a heart attack or a perforated stomach, it's reasonable to act on that possibility because it's so bad to delay you were wrong. The more serious the consequences of being wrong, the more those slender possibilities become reasonable to consider. ☼

But deciding to run one more test based on that "one in a million" possibility is not "reasonable." That type of

221

practice is called "Defensive Medicine" and it raises the cost of healthcare for everybody without getting people healthier.

WE HAVE TO GET THE BULLET OUT!!!

In movies, no matter what, when the hero is shot and for some reason they can't take him/ her to the hospital, they find someone who can dig out the bullet.

In Hollywood, if you can remove the bullet, the subject recovers. So they stick something through the bullet hole, even their fingers, root around a little, roll their eyes, finally find the bullet and then place it in a cup where it lands with a satisfying "clunk."

Oh hooray, he's going to live!

In real life, you can leave the bullet in. Often it would cause more damage to remove it. Depending on the location, you need to operate to repair critical damage caused by the bullet such as a torn, bleeding artery. You close up holes in lungs which cause them to collapse and not re-inflate until repaired. You sew over holes in intestines that would pollute the entire abdominal cavity and result in severe infections.

The corollary to this Hollywood nonsense is that if the movie bullet passes through, it's a clean wound and nothing needs to be done.

Does everyone in Tinseltown think the audience has no doctors, nurses, surgical techs, or even knowledgeable lay people who pay attention to the world?

Every time this happens in a show my wife and I are watching at home, I yell out, "Getting the bullet out is irrelevant!!" And my wife responds, "Quiet! It's only a movie!"

The Patient's Values Affect the Reasonableness of What Is Possible

In the patient with the gastro-colic fistula, it would have been reasonable to test for that even if there had been only one chance in 100 she had something like that. That was a problem from which the patient could have survived only with surgery. She would have died if the diagnosis were missed. This cocky surgeon did not know her. He made assumptions.

Even if he had been right in the assumption that a reasonable physician would conclude this patient was probably only seeking drugs, it would not excuse his negligence. Even with a one in 100 possibility that she was truly sick, it was necessary to work her up for that possibility.

When I gave her enough time to report "bad-smelling vomit" the odds of finding a deadly problem were much higher. But he did not ask enough questions to get that far.

I used to tell my students: If you listen long enough to your patients, they might tell you what's wrong with them. ☼

Suppose you have chest pain and the Myocardial Infarction Risk Calculator (based on your cholesterol, systolic blood pressure, and age) says your risk of a heart attack that year is only 1%.

Here's how we doctors should think it through. We estimate a 1% possibility of the chest pain representing a heart attack. We realize there is very good treatment available for a heart attack. We realize that delay in treatment of a heart attack can have adverse consequences for the patient. Finally, we might ask ourselves "Would it be a bad thing to bring 100 patients to the hospital to prevent one from dying or if not dying, surviving with a permanently weakened heart?"

These illustrations are not absolute or exact. You can't just look them up the odds of everything. Doctors can make a rough estimate though. What's more, the value to the patient of the different possibilities must be considered.

"Not dying" sounds like a value that everyone would go for. But every patient has different circumstances. For a 50-year-old patient with chest pain at 3 a.m. and a one in 100 possibility of having a heart attack, the best choice might be "Let's go to the hospital," In contrast, the 98-year-old patient who's pain was tolerable might choose to say, "That's OK, I'll stay home and try an antacid."

I am not suggesting we should treat patients less cautiously due to their age. I'm saying, try to find out, "How do the values of the patient affect the decision?"

I'm suggesting that the patient at age 98 might fear death less than the 50-year-old. I am suggesting that a wise, well-informed patient at age 98 might decide to go with the flow rather than pursue invasive treatments. The decision might be different for a 50-year-old in the final stages of terminal cancer. At that point, the patient may choose to stay in bed and take an antacid, even with a 1 in 10 risk of heart attack versus indigestion. Since delay could result in the death of more heart muscle during a heart attack, that should be unthinkable for the patient without a terminal illness.

Ultimately decision-making should be based on the patient's value system. A doctor should not willingly put himself/herself in the role of making a value decision without input from the patient. Otherwise, we will look at the situation through the lens of the doctor's values and never learn the patient's values.

I think a good doctor explores the patient's values when the patient is making what seems to be an unreasonable decision. You might find out the patient would want to follow reasonable advice except for "who's going to watch my dog?" or "We have tickets for a cruise in two days."

Maybe it is time to define value. Value is Benefit divided by Cost. In shopping, a good value is a good product divided by a low cost. A Rolls Royce is a very expensive good product and may offer great benefits in certain circles, but the cost of one is very, very high, like $400,000. The benefits of a Rolls are not that much greater than our usual vehicle. So when you consider the benefit/cost, the Rolls is not a good value. You know this math, now apply it to medical decisions.

Let your doctor know about your "values." If you have always been worried about cancer and lots of family members had cancer yet the doctor says the odds of cancer are only one in 500 and that still bugs you, then maybe you should ask about getting that test anyway. It would have a high value to you. It might not be reasonable for someone else. You need to hope your insurance won't deny the claim for the test. They might deny it if their guideline book suggests the cancer concern in your situation is not a "reasonable" one or if early detection is not useful for that cancer. Then the benefit, in their eyes, is small compared to the cost.

If there is time, research what respected guidelines and medical journal editorials recommend, realizing that the medical profession can be slow to adapt to change. Consider doing nothing if there is no serious downside. Consider your values and realize that even good doctors may find it easier to use their personal values over your values if you have not slowed down their rushed thinking to give them time to input your values into their mental calculatioins. Ask your doctor to sit down and then start asking your questions.

It's Not Like an Election

I used to explain to my medical students that when a slender possibility wins out over a likely probability it's because medical decision-making is not like voting in an election.

In political elections, the candidate with the most votes wins. In a two-person race, it's 50% plus one vote to win.

In medicine, when weighing possible outcomes of your potentially life-altering decision, the "winner of the election" is the possibility with the most serious outcome if you fail to consider it.

Three Blind Mice?

In our basement we have four mousetraps all in a row, in a crawl space, about four inches apart. Twenty-nine days out of 30 we catch no mice. One day we caught three. I wondered what the second and third mice were thinking when they saw the first mouse dead in the trap and decided to throw caution to the wind and nibble on the bait in the other two traps anyway. How bizarre really. It's like with smokers. What do smokers think when they have seen other smokers dying from smoking-related illnesses and yet they put the next cigarette in their mouth?

A Simple Decision Matrix for an Actual Patient with Chest Pain at 3 a.m.

I am using chest pain to illustrate decision-making. If you are too young to worry about your heart, this chapter may be of use to you regardless. You may want to use a decision matrix when you consider whether to wear a helmet on your cycle.

Years ago, I knew a 60-year-old physician who developed chest pain at 3 a.m. He waited until 7 a.m. to call the ambulance. When the symptom began, a clot had formed in one of the coronary arteries that supplies fresh blood to the heart muscle. We believe a clot like that is the fundamental cause of a heart attack. The clot blocks the delivery of oxygen-rich blood to the heart muscle, which then gradually starts to die.

Similarly, a clot in the brain can deprive oxygen to a part of the brain causing a stroke. Brain tissue dies easily and much faster during a stroke compared with heart muscle dying in a heart attack.

Heart muscle with very low oxygen due to a blocked blood supply takes hours to complete the death process. That means if the blood were restored in a few hours, the heart muscle at risk can be brought back. Yes, that's worth repeating: If the blood flow is restored within the first few hours, the heart muscle affected by the heart attack can recover!

If the heart attack is not reversed, that portion of the heart turns into a scar that won't squeeze with the rest of the heart.

For this 60-year-old doctor, who delayed four hours before calling the ambulance, his heart's artery would not be restored (revascularized). The affected heart muscle was permanently damaged and the heart was left in a weakened state for the rest of his life. The doctor needed treatment for heart failure.

Why did he delay? He said, "I thought it was indigestion." In truth, he knew it could have been a heart attack. The most likely probability (over 50% likely) was indigestion. But the narrower possibility, maybe 10%, in his case, was a heart attack. Why did he not act in the best way to preserve his own heart? I have seen this type of thinking error among both doctors and patients more times than I care to recall.

With experience, you don't need to plot out this kind of matrix to solve every problem, but a decision matrix like this one helps illustrate the options for critical decisions and leads you to you the better choices.

Decision matrix for a sixty year old waking up with chest pain at 3 a.m.

Possibilities (possible cause of the chest and pain)	Likelihood or Probability	Consequence of delay	Priority	Action
Indigestion	High, over 50%	None	Low	Taken an antacid and wait
Heart Attack	Lower, maybe 10%	Death or permanent heart failure	High	Call ambulance and go to hospital

In medicine, temporizing means giving the situation some time before acting, to see if the problem will go away on its own. Temporizing is a useful tool because many things do go away.

We can get fooled a lot by reviewing our experiences rather than using the logic of the matrix. If the doctor treats the condition based on the most likely probability and the patient gets better, the patient will give credit to the treatment and the doctor feels he did the right thing. For example: Let's pretend our 60-year-old physician-patient had called his doctor at 3 a.m. and the last six times his patients had nighttime chest pain, the doctor had recommended an antacid for "waking up with indigestion at night," and if none of those patients turned out to have had heart attacks, the doctor might figure out that he was pretty smart. He might have patted himself on the back for helping his patients avoid an expensive and uncomfortable ambulance ride and ER visit. But look at the matrix and you can see he would have been wrong.

This type of error of thinking is akin to deciding what to do on the basis of anecdotes, as discussed earlier. Anecdotes don't prove the case.

Look at the item in the box on the "Heart Attack" row and the Consequence of Delay column. It says, "Death or permanent heart failure."

That's the entry that determines the right decision. If in another case it said, "No harm" to delay, it would be fine to wait.

Doctors are sometimes criticized for charging a fee when not "doing" anything. But we have to acknowledge that the body has a lot of ways of healing itself and we need to treat that patient the best way, even if the educated choice to do nothing leads to lower satisfaction scores.

In my first practice we were hiring a new doctor. During an interview, I asked him, "What do you do if a patient comes in with a viral illness like a cold."

He replied that he prescribed an antibiotic because if he didn't, the patient wouldn't be happy.

For this reason, we did not hire him.

If all the possible outcomes that would result from the various choices are comparatively innocent, choose the action which corresponds with the most likely possibility. Take the antacid and wait to see if you feel better. If one of the possibilities is potentially lethal like maybe it's a heart attack, forget the probabilities, favor that unacceptable possibility, and call 911.

If you are too young to worry about heart attacks think of this example. "I have driven my motorcycle 100s of times without an accident so I don't need a helmet." Can you draw the matrix for this decision? Clue: the second row reads: Possibility: Accident Resulting in Brain injury/ Likelihood low/ Consequence: Brain damage, being a vegetable, rest of your life in a nursing home/ Action: Wear helmet.

This sounds like the most obvious common sense but in my career, I saw doctors and patients break this rule all the time.

Picture Windows, Christmas Trees, and a Back Stretching Testimonial

My patient had back problems, like a lot of patients. He lived in an area between towns north of us. In other words, he lived out in the country. I try to keep patient details obscured. Let's call him Jack since that was not his name.

Jack told me about his neighbor Fred who grew Christmas trees. That holiday season, we gave up searching for the right tree from the collections of cut trees sold on parking lots around town and we drove to Fred's tree farm. Fred eventually became my patient too.

If not for the tree farm, I probably would have never seen Jack's home. It was located in what we suburbanites call the middle of nowhere.

From Jack and other country-dwelling patients, I had learned that one of the economies of living in an uncrowned rural neighborhood is that you may not need to buy blinds or curtains for every window. In suburbia, you need window coverings for privacy. But in the country, according to some people whose homes are sufficiently isolated, there is not enough traffic passing by to justify the purchase of window blinds in every window.

Not everybody likes being in the open country. When my wife and I lived in northern Arizona at 5000 feet elevation, we saw a lot of open land for sure. One day, driving on a deserted highway, I could see mountain ranges on either side of the road 10 to 20 miles away and we could see a small village five miles ahead. I said to my wife, "Isn't it peaceful out here?" She said, "Peaceful? You mean desolated!"

Back to my story in Ohio. Each December on the way to Fred's farm for our Christmas Tree, we would pass by Jack's house. Jack had a huge picture window facing the

231

road. That was the one Jack told me had no curtains or blinds.

Jack had muscular back problems. I had told him to do frequent but brief back stretches for maybe 20 seconds all through the day, in fact, every time he thought of it.

Reader, try this now. Stand up. Slowly bend a little to the left then to the right, then forward a little and then backward. Do it again.

Now sit down and keep reading. I don't know about you but my back feels better. For the back, immobility sucks.☼

I'll tell you what happened the way Jack told me. One of his other neighbors was coming home from a bar at 1 a.m. and he saw Jack through that front picture window doing his back exercises. The neighbor thought that the middle of the night was a strange time to do back exercises. The next time they met, he said "Jack why were you doing your stretches at 1 a.m.?

Jack told me, "I said I got up to use the bathroom and I do my back stretches every time I think about them because they make my back feel better. So that's why."

This is what you call an unsolicited testimonial.

A Short Primer on Sore Backs and Soup

A lot of knowledge in practice comes from the ideas and observations of patients. They give you clues and help you form theories. The theory here is that back stretching helps people with back pain. After forming a theory, someone has to perform research to prove the point to medical science

But some harmless and "free" stuff like the back stretches I recommend are so benign that sometimes a doctor just advises patients based on what works.

I prescribed stretching exercises because it helped people feel better when muscular back strains were healing. I did not advise them because of studies. I am sure that plenty of studies on stretching have been published, after being generously funded and influenced by the evil lords of the back stretching industry I'm sure. But how do you set up a control group to compare the stretching group with the non-stretchers? I just didn't look for those studies.

Let's contrast back stretches with laser treatments for sore back muscles. Should a doctor prescribe twenty $300 laser treatments (cost $6000) because they "seem" to work? No way.

Because of that big cost, the idea that back laser treatment should replace or even be added to back stretches needs to be proven before patients in the US spend $Billions on that theory.

I will confess that I liked it when patients returned and said their back felt better. I especially got a chuckle when they had failed to improve with pills before getting my advice to do the stretches. To get patients to do those exercises I had to explain it in some way. I used an analogy.

I'd say to my patient: Let's say you want to make some soup, cooking it for hours on the stove.

Which would be smarter? Option 1: Stir the soup constantly for 20 minutes and then leave it untouched on the stove for four hours, or Option 2: Stir the soup for 10 to 20 seconds every 15 minutes?

Everybody gets the right answer: you have to keep stirring the soup or it will stick to the pot or even burn.

I would explain that it is the same with back problems. Don't perform stretching exercises one time a day in the morning for 20 minutes and then sit at your desk, the back nearly immobilized the rest of the day.

No, you need to move your back every ten minutes: flex forward just a little, to the left just a little, to the right just a little. It is very important to perform extension which is the opposite of flexion. You push out your belly or your chest, leaning your head back. That extends the lumbar spine. You can do this in a chair. You can do it in a meeting. Don't go so far that it hurts and if any motion hurts, see a doctor.

Many patients won't follow this simple advice. If they walk and stand all day they think their back is getting moved enough. But when they walk or stand they are not bending to the sides or extending.

Doctors tend to dislike treating backs because medicines are ineffective. If I did not find reasons to suspect something more serious like a herniated disc or infection or kidney stone or aortic aneurysm, I found that it's worthwhile to try stretching exercises. That advice frequently worked.

Here's a fact about backs that is still "behind the curtain" for many patients. Back surgery does not help sore backs. ☼

Rather, back surgery is useful to decompress lumbar nerve roots that are being rubbed or squeezed by abnormal things in the spine such as herniated discs or bone spurs. The lumbar nerve roots form from the spinal nerves and go down to supply your thighs, legs, and feet. Decompression means taking the pressure off.

The surgery can help with pain or weakness in the thigh and below. It won't help the back muscles. Even after back surgery, you need mobilization exercises to take away back pain.

So if you just have back pain without the numbness or weakness of the thighs and legs, don't worry about surgery. See your doctor to rule out the bad stuff. If you have pain down the thigh or the leg, the doctor will have to think about a lumbar disc or other structure pushing on the lumbar nerve root that supplies the thigh, leg, or foot.

As I mentioned, low back pain rarely could be caused by an expanding aortic aneurysm. Back pain with fever can be caused by a spinal abscess. Back pain worse in the middle of the night could be caused by a tumor in the spine. Back pain on only one side could be caused by a kidney stone, so see the doctor if you have some unusual or severe or new back issue.

"I Am Not In the Information Business, I Am in the Hope Business."

Once I moderated an online discussion about the ethics of cancer treatment. Over 100 doctors participated. I created a hypothetical case to facilitate the discussion. The patient was a man in his 40s with a cancer that could be treated but not all that well. The best to hope for with treatment was that 10% of the patients would live two years. Ninety percent of those treated did not respond and lived only one year, the same as the one year survival for those who opted to receive no treatment. But the longer survival would mean living two years with pain and chemotherapy side effects. The patients with no treatment would have no pain for six months and pain from the disease for the last six months. The 90% who did not respond to treatment would have side effects of chemotherapy and then pain from the tumor and then die in 12 months. Now his life was pretty OK except for knowing he had cancer.

Some doctors call treatment in a case like this one an attempt to "prolong the patient's life" but other doctors who struggle with the notion of futile medical care favor calling it "prolonging the patient's death."

Even worse, the patient in the scenario had no health insurance. Aggressive treatment would result in huge out-of-pocket expenses, about $300,000 consuming the spouse's equity in their home as well as all they had saved for their child's college fund, which had not been protected by being invested in a state college saving program.

The question I posed to the doctors in the online discussion group was whether the oncologist should present all the options and the details of the financial cost as well as the percentage of patients who would get various outcomes: the numbers I provided above.

Should the oncologist say something like, "This treatment might cost $300,000. I am sorry to tell you the effectiveness of what we can do for you is disappointing. For every 100 people like you, with treatment about 10 will live two years. The rest of the treated patients will on average die in a year. Without treatment on average patients last one year. But those are averages. Your results could vary. You could live only three months with treatment if you suffered severe side effects. Or you could get extremely lucky and survive six years but the odds of that are 1 in 1000. On average you would have a 10% of surviving an extra year with treatment."

In my experience, some of my cancer patients with very terrible cancers with a similarly bad future would come back to see me after seeing the oncologist the first time and say, "Well, the oncologist and I discussed the treatment and it's very serious but I'm going to have radiation, surgery, and chemotherapy. The results of treatment for my tumor have been improving. I'm hopeful."

I would leave the exam room with a bad taste in my mouth. The oncologist only told them the positive side. Results are improving? How many out of 100 in the trials? I worried that my patient had been manipulated by receiving an incomplete set of truths.

Most of the other doctors in the online discussion were primary care doctors like me and they shared my experiences and my frustrations. Some of the doctors made some fairly insulting comments about oncologists being biased by huge profits from chemotherapy, which they could earn in those days.

One oncologist in the online group defended the progress being made in chemotherapy. And the question was asked of him by the others, shouldn't we offer accurate statistics of success v failure before the patient is treated? Don't patients need this information?

He responded curtly: "I am in the hope business, not the information business."

Next I will to discuss what it is to be professional in one's field.

Professionalism

When I became Vice President of Medical Affairs, at the first medical staff executive committee meeting of the academic year, I welcomed the new president of the medical staff. I commended his professionalism and offered an expanded definition of that term.

Professionalism: practicing an art with efficiency or skill or high quality...and with subordination of self interest. Deemphasizing self-interest is another aspect to professionalism, which is not always thought of in the definition of the word.

Professionals are driven by an internal obligation to put the needs of the client, known as the patient in our profession, and the needs of society above their personal interests and benefit.

We need to teach this concept to our medical students.

A Professional Sense of Obligation to Reveal Absolute Differences Not Just the Relative Comparison.

What's an internal obligation?

That means the driving desire to favor the interests of the patient is part of the intrinsic nature of the doctor. It is not something being forced upon him/her by some external authority or rule.

I remember a friend who told me he hired a bricklayer to lay his patio. The man worked for a big contractor on weekdays, but on weekends he worked for himself. He did a marvelous job for my friend. The bricks were arranged in a striking herringbone pattern. The bricklayer explained he loved doing these side jobs. He said on his weekday job he had to slow down his pace to match his co-workers. Otherwise, they would resent him for finishing too soon and making them look bad. Herringbone and other patterns were rarely done because the company charged a premium fee for that type of brickwork. But for his weekend clients, he could let loose his natural speed and his exacting geometric creativity.

By my way of looking at things, that bricklayer was a professional. I described an expanded definition of professionalism above. Professionals are driven by an internal obligation to put the needs of the client (known as the patient in our profession) and the needs of society above their personal interests and benefit.

I will tell a story about a medical conference to illustrate what I would call unprofessional bias and data manipulation.

Most hospitals have tumor conferences. These are not hypothetical cases like my online discussion group. At these conferences, the doctors present the cases of real cancer patients. Doctors in the several specialties that treat cancer

239

will give their opinions as to how that patient should be treated. The radiation oncologists discuss what their therapy could offer, the medical oncologists discuss their approach to chemotherapy, the cancer surgeons discuss the effectiveness of surgery and the primary care doctors usually sip their coffee and learn. That's how our tumor conferences went.

This tumor conference was more than 25 years ago. I am being a bit inaccurate to hide the doctors involved, because the people in the story don't matter. I am critical of the behaviors.

One patient had a truly awful type of cancer. The surgeon and the radiation oncologist spoke about the limited options for this tumor.

Their treatments would not offer much to help the patient with that diagnosis. Nothing would.

Then the medical oncologist stood up. He objected to the negative attitude of the other doctors and proposed treatment with chemotherapy. I will always remember what he said: "The five-year survival numbers are 100% better now than five years ago." His authority won over the conference members.

At the end of that day, I checked a new online reference that I had discovered in those early days of the internet. It was the National Cancer Institute (NCI) internet site. I looked up the treatment for this cancer.

My confident colleague, the oncologist, was right, sort of. The five-year survival was indeed 100% improved. But a few years ago the chemo helped just one in 200 patients live five years and now it could help two in 200 patients. Going from one to two is indeed a 100% improvement in relative terms. But in absolute terms, chemo was helping only one additional patient out of 200 - not much of a benefit.

Pay close attention to that man behind the curtain who tries to impress you with **relative** benefit without stating the **absolute** benefit. Relative benefit: 100% improvement. Absolute benefit: one in 200. Mentioning the one without the other seems like manipulation to me. ☼

Here's an example. You are told a new treatment is 50% better than the old one. You need to ask for the absolute figures. Does that mean it used to help 20% of the patients and now it helps 30%? Does it mean it used to help 2% of the patients and now it helps 3%? There's a big difference!

In my opinion, the doctor who is a "professional" will mention both absolute and relative improvement data. If someone in the medical field offers you a relative comparison ask for the absolute figures.

Facts Rejected - Hope Wins - Patient Loses

I am not against doctors offering patients a long shot. It's OK with me to treat 100 people inflicted with an awful disease even if you can only save one. It's OK by me to treat all 100 just to help the one who wouldn't survive. I'm not against the 99 who suffered through treatment and die regardless. It's all OK if that's what the patients wanted. This is an issue of patient rights. I just think the patients need to know these statistics before they agree to the tests or treatments being proposed.

I remember a nice older lady who always came to my office with her retired husband. They were in their mid-70s.

I can remember them very well even though it was over 30 years ago. I discovered that she had a type of bladder cancer that was different from the most common type which is highly curable. Hers was invasive and highly aggressive.

I was one of the first doctors in my circle who had Internet access. The Internet was new and we didn't yet have the World Wide Web, which dates to 1991.

I was on the volunteer staff of the local medical school which had begun offering online access to the faculty. I signed up so early that my user name was two letters, RS. Later they figured out they should reserve the two-digit user names for the "Big Kahunas" at the med school. I was not in that category. I was just among the first to sign up. I only mention these details to show that internet access was unusual then.

The Internet was a black screen with green characters like in the movie War Games. There was no search engine such as Google or Duck Duck Go. Somehow I found a site called PDQ. PDQ to me had meant "pretty damn quick" but this stood for "Physician Data Query. It was under the NIH's NCI, the National Institutes of Health's National Cancer Institute.

This site amazed me. You didn't have to wait for the patient to see the oncologist and then wait for a letter. You didn't need to buy a $200 textbook of oncology that was out of date the month after it was published. You could look up and read about the latest treatments and outcomes for all kinds of cancers!

My patient didn't ask me to do this research. I just did it because her type of aggressive bladder cancer was something I had not seen before. She was going to need my advice on whether she should be treated locally or at a tertiary care center. We were a little more than an hour away from the Cleveland Clinic. I had found that although the Cleveland Clinic did very well with unusual diseases, it didn't stand above other hospitals in the treatment of ordinary conditions or untreatable conditions.

I looked up the treatment and prognosis for my patient's type of aggressive bladder cancer. It became evident to me the patient's prognosis was very poor with or without treatment. It was unlikely she was going to live more than six months either way.

Treatment would be an exercise in futility. It would provide suffering with negligible chance of prolonged survival.

At her next visit a few days later, I explained this sad prognosis to the patient and to her husband. She wasn't having a lot of symptoms yet and I advised her to enjoy the next few months of her life and delay treatment. It was time to do things on the "Bucket List."

She couldn't accept my advice. Maybe it was because I was merely a family doctor. Maybe it was because patients seem to be brainwashed with the notion that early treatment always improves the outcome of cancer. That's only true for some cancers.

She referred herself to the Cleveland Clinic where she underwent extremely aggressive cancer surgery followed by chemotherapy. She endured serious complications. In three months she was dead as a result of these complications, having suffered most of that time.

What Informed Consent did she receive at the Cleveland Clinic? I don't know. Nowadays the laws outline the right of the patient to Informed Consent. Here's how those rights are explained on the American Cancer Website with my comment in bold.

Informed consent is a process of communication between you and your health care provider that often leads to agreement or permission for care, treatment, or services. Every patient has the right to get information and ask questions before procedures and treatments. If adult patients are mentally able to make their own decisions, medical care cannot begin unless they give informed consent.

The informed consent process makes sure that your health care provider has given you information about your condition along with testing and treatment options before you decide what to do.

[NOTE it does not require "complete" information or "balanced" presentations or "Pros and Cons" or require meaningful statistics such as absolute v relative benefit in comparing options]

This information can include:

- The name of your condition
- The name of the procedure or treatment that the health care provider recommends
- Risks and benefits of the treatment or procedure
- Risks and benefits of other options, including not getting the treatment or procedure

Signing informed consent means

- You have received all the information about your treatment options from your health care provider.
- You understand the information and you have had a chance to ask questions.
- You use this information to decide if you want to receive the recommended treatment option(s) that have been explained to you. Sometimes, you may choose to receive only part of the recommended care. Talk to your health care provider about your options.
- If you agree to receive all or some of the treatment options, you give your consent (agree) by signing a consent form. The completed and signed form is a legal document that lets your doctor go ahead with the treatment plan.

If you had a procedure done in the United States in the last decade did you get all this information about options, benefits and risks?

You have the right to information! But you need to ask pointed questions to fully realize the benefits of this right. Think twice before you sign the consent form the doctor's assistant brings to you when you haven't had the chance to finish quizzing the doctor. You don't want to make critical decisions about your life based on only *some* of the alternative options and only some of the information about those options.

Bias of Online Materials and Prejudices

Sometimes we fail when trying to do the right thing. Emotional thinking has a stronger pull than logical reasoning. Prejudices may affect us in ways we don't realize.

We have discussed physician bias based on the physician's self-interest and based on pride. I want to go over bias on the Internet and also prejudices.

Some of us have an idea that if the doctor doesn't have time to talk to us, we can find the answer on the Internet, right?

Yes, information online is available, boy is it ever, if you're willing to wade through it, but you may find so many different versions of the truth your head will spin.

Which is the most correct answer? Which version of the online truth is the one we should rely on before making a decision on which our health or even our life may depend?

Paying close attention to that man behind the curtain in this case means being alert for bias. Look for conflicts of interest. What's best for you, the patient, as opposed to what's good for the person who composed the content you found on the internet?

There are two general kinds of bias: Explicit and Implicit.

Explicit bias is conscious. The person holding the bias is or should be aware of their bias. It is not a surprise to them and it should not be a surprise to you that they favor certain attitudes or proposed courses of action. Often there is a financial payoff involved or to put it another way, more income for them.

The person listening to the biased persuasion should be able to recognize the conflict of interest unless the financial relationships are hidden. You shouldn't be surprised or even disappointed if a surgeon recommends surgery if the decision is medical v. surgical. I am not saying surgeons are incapable of subordinating their self-interest. But if it's a toss-up, the surgeon might recommend surgery.

You shouldn't be surprised if sites that are selling a medication favor the product sold by the company that put up the website.

I remember being in the office of an older family doctor before the Internet. A drug salesman popped in to make a quick presentation of a new product. His talk was short, factual, and persuasive. It was also TOTALLY biased. When he finished the salesman asked what the old doctor thought of this new drug. Getting up from his chair and walking past the salesman on his way to the next patient, the senior doctor simply mumbled, "Based on what you just told me, I think this must be the best drug ever invented."

That was a great backhanded complement. It was like saying of a politician "if being charming means being narcissistic, bombastic, ignorant, prejudiced, inconsistent, and dishonest, he is the most charming politician around."

Sometimes the patient does not see the explicit nature of the bias. Do the patients know if the person who wrote what they read on the internet profits from the stuff they are recommending?

You should not get angry about explicit bias. You're just wasting energy.

I like telling the story about the good-natured fellow who was watching a wounded rattler try to cross the highway. From the looks of it, a truck must have run over the poor snake's tail.

The man grabbed a long stick and used it to pick up the snake and help it to the other side of the road. Once there, the snake struck him. "Why did you bite me?" he cried. The snake replied, "Don't act surprised! You knew I was a snake! This is what I do."

Often when getting medical information from the Internet we don't recognize the explicit bias until 30 clicks later when the commercialism is revealed. After spending 20 minutes and clicking "NEXT" again and again, and becoming more and more curious about this marvelous advance in medicine we have been seduced to click on, suddenly the "order page" appears. You can get your first bottle for $10 compared to the usual price of $150. "Don't you know what a good deal this is? Buy now!" Yep, that spiel might just be biased, don't you think?

No, don't get upset about explicit bias. It's predictable.

The second type of bias is implicit bias. That type is subconscious and has to do with thoughts and principles which are ingrained in the biased writer. The person with implicit bias may be unaware of how it affects him/ her.

A lot of what people call prejudice fits into the category of implicit bias.

Misogyny is often ingrained. For example, for years it has been recognized that physicians are less likely to consider the diagnosis of ischemic heart disease in women. Black patients are less likely to receive aggressive cancer treatments. In both situations, the problem is probably implicit bias.

How can a person not realize they are biased? Bias against women is ingrained in a lot of us. Here's a little riddle you may have heard.

One day, a father and his son were driving in the same car and suffered a serious motor vehicle collision. They were midway between two hospitals. They were both critically injured. Ambulances arrived on the scene. The father was taken to the hospital five miles to the north and the boy to the one five miles to the south. When the boy arrived at Emergency, the ER doctor immediately called the surgeon on duty. The surgeon walked in and said, "Oh my God, it's my son."

Can you explain?

This is an old joke but I felt a little bad when so many liberated women, even women physicians respond, "The other man was his stepfather." Or, "The boy was adopted." But the simplest explanation is that surgeon is the boy's *mother*.

The assumption that surgeons are men is an ingrained attitude that is finally changing. It is not a conscious bias, it is an implicit bias.

I mentioned that we sometimes have trouble ferreting out implicit bias in ourselves. Healthcare professionals hold the same implicit biases as the general population. Assumptions are made on the basis of the patient's skin color or country of origin or religion.

I have seen Black patients who told me they wanted to go to Caucasian doctors. They were biased against Black physicians. The patient does not admit to that prejudice but it's part of their makeup. That's implicit bias.

If you come to the doctor's visit wearing your best clean clothes you may fit into a positive bias. What if you come to the office smelling like cigarettes or dirty clothes? You can fix that. What if you are not college-educated? If you're not well educated, maybe bring a friend who is. What if you are poor? What if you are well-to-do? I have seen doctors with bias against wealthy patients.

If something triggers an implicit bias in your doctor, you may not recognize it and neither may your doctor recognize it. It is more important than ever to research your treatment options before you see your doctor and then discuss them with him/her. The doctor may have a bias in favor of being very thorough with patients who have done their homework.

Know Everything About Nothing

Not enough people have a broad base of layman's medical knowledge to aid in medical decision-making.

Today we live in an age of hyperspecialization and that's not just among doctors. The broad education required to earn a college degree is being replaced by an ever more narrow focus or specialization. Engineers have minimal exposure to language arts. Literature and history majors have minimal exposure to the sciences.

I think doctors should have more experience in subjects outside of science. The aspiring medical student can easily escape the study of history, government, ethics, social sciences, literature, and world cultures. Most pre-medical students major in sciences.

I was fortunate to have majored in English literature. Most people think I must have been an oddball to have done that. Yet I believe studying language and literature has been a major help to my career. I confess I probably was an oddball but I became less of one for having a college major outside of the sciences.

The other Dr. Sinsheimer in the family, my younger son, is a physicist at a research lab. He spent six years in physics graduate school to get his Ph.D. after four years in college. Then he did two post-doctoral studies. When he was in graduate school he told me, "As a person becomes more educated, he learns more and more about less and less until eventually, he knows everything about nothing."

There is overspecialization outside of medicine and science too. We had an estimate to replace our concrete drive and the contractor said he could not replace the concrete front porch. We needed a different type of concrete guy for that.

249

I recall a patient who had finished six years with the Air Force and was now looking for a job. He told me he had been a jet plane mechanic in the service. I told him I thought airplane mechanics might be a good field for him. But he said he would never be able to find work as an airplane mechanic. He had been too highly specialized. His skill was that he removed one panel on one side of one kind of jet fighter and serviced what was inside that panel. He had no training on how to service the opposite side of the plane, or the nose section, the tail, the gears, the canopy, the avionics, the weapons, the radar or the engines, or anything on a different jet.

I had another patient who spent six years in Japan as a missionary and came back to the States. He was unsuccessfully looking for a job to support his large family. I asked him why he did not capitalize on his knowledge of the Japanese language? Surely a good career and income could evolve out of that language skill, right? At that time, Japan was the world's fastest-growing economy and the Japanese were buying American businesses and properties. They needed Americans who spoke Japanese.

No, he told me, his Japanese was limited to the sort of words used in the effort to convert the Japanese to Christianity. He was a specialist in converting non-Christians. In the fields of business or real estate or manufacturing, his Japanese was useless to a potential employer.

Those patients had to learn something new to get good jobs. The antidote to the lack of general knowledge in our population is a lifetime of self-study. Benjamin Franklin was a man of extremely broad learning. He was enrolled in a school from age eight to age ten. That was it! But he read extensively all his life. He founded one of the first libraries in this country and helped found the University of Pennsylvania.

You should include some science and medicine among your topics for self-study. Perhaps this book would be a start for you.

You Can Gather Enough Knowledge of Your Condition to Phrase the Best Questions.

More and more people know nothing about so many things. If we are going to make decisions with patients, we need patients to have enough general knowledge of medicine to come up with the right questions to ask. In some situations, they may need to study issues they would never have needed to know about before.

A man goes into a doctor's office and goes up to the window. "Can I have an appointment today?" he asks. The receptionist looks at the schedule and shakes her head, "I'm sorry the doctor has no appointments for today, how about two tomorrow?" The patient looks surprised. "Oh, no, I just want one appointment."

If you are young or speeding reading, the preceding paragraph is known as a "Dad Joke."

Two appointments? If you think your questions will require a lot of time, let the scheduler know. Maybe you do need two appointment slots. The doctor is often rushed. If there was no time during this visit to compose your ideas and formulate good questions that matter to you, make another appointment to discuss your questions in greater depth. Make it clear when scheduling that this visit is for this one purpose. Doctors have to charge based on a codebook and there are ways to charge for counseling, which is what this would be.

How can I ask the doctor a good question if I'm way over my head?

Once you get past the vocabulary, medicine is not that intellectually daunting compared with a lot of other fields. We make it seem difficult by using a lot of jargon, or words that are well understood by medical people but difficult for others. "Doctor talk." Learning some doctor talk helps. In most cases, ordinary English works fine.

I always tried to talk in plain English and was amused when patients would fire back using medical jargon.

I would ask, "Do you get out of breath when you shouldn't?"

"Yes, doctor, I have mild to moderate dyspnea."

"Do you have pain in the lower part of your belly?"

"Yes, I have some right lower quadrant pain."

Some common English words have specific meanings in the world of medicine. I must confess I get picky over arm v. forearm and leg v. thigh.

The words "leg" and "arm" are misused. I want to know what the patient means.

Technically the thigh is the part between the hip and the knee and the part between the knee and the ankle is the leg. The arm is the section between the shoulder and the elbow and the part between the elbow and the wrist is the forearm. When someone says I have a problem in my leg I always need to clarify what they mean. Is the "upper leg" the thigh or do they mean the part between the mid calf and the knee?

Most medical knowledge is not over-complex. In contrast, my son in physics works in a difficult-to-comprehend field. They experiment with high-energy beams of light and x-ray. I remember how my wife's cousin told us he enjoyed talking to him at the family reunion.

He said, "Your son told me about his research and it was interesting to hear him describe it, but I have to confess I got lost after the word 'The'."

But medicine is comparatively lightweight stuff, intellectually. You need to know the prostate from the pancreas and things like that.

Sometimes your science background helps you understand concepts. For example, someone tells you that tomatoes are acidic. You shouldn't eat them because you have a history of ulcers.

Is that good advice? You don't need to be a doctor to figure this out. Googling tells you the stomach acid has a pH of 2 and tomatoes have a pH of 4. You look up the pH scale. A pH of 4 is 1/10 as strong as pH 3 which is 1/10 as strong as pH of 2. So if the tomato is two pH steps down, it is only 1/100 as acidic as stomach acid. Tomatoes are not going to burn your stomach.

Regardless tomatoes can *upset* stomachs, but it's not their weak acidity. It's something about how an individual reacts to tomatoes.

If the doctor explains that to you, and you have no education in simple chemistry and physics, you might get lost after the word "The."

A person with a broad general education can figure out a lot these days if motivated to do the research. Everyone has holes in their knowledge base.

Growing vegetables is a weak area for me. Once I tried to grow corn without fertilizer. I grew such tiny ears of corn!

But I can learn. I want to show you how to learn and figure out things: One summer I grew tomatoes in pots. I used the internet to choose a good hybrid with a reputation for disease resistance and for excellent taste. I started the seedlings indoors for three weeks in April.

I used the Internet to find out when it was safe to put the pots outside overnight, after the last freeze. The first tomatoes came and all developed soft brown spots on the lower part of the fruit. I Googled "tomatoes with soft brown bottoms." I found the problem was something called "blossom-end rot" and it was due to calcium deficiency. I found you could buy calcium plant supplements to remedy the problem. I was too lazy to go to the store.

I also learned online that Tums (which contains calcium carbonate) might help tomatoes. We had some Tums in the medicine closet. My general knowledge of the world told me the calcium carbonate was chalk, like the stuff which make up the White Cliffs of Dover. It turns out that calcium carbonate dissolves poorly in water. That rings true. Otherwise, the White Cliffs would melt every time it rained in England and the chalk would have run into the English Channel eons ago.

I found the Tums and crushed a few of them into powder and added water in a measuring cup to make a slurry.

I knew the crushed Tums tablet was not going to dissolve but crushed it would release more calcium than the intact tablet.

That would be a function of the surface area exposed to the water. With that in mind, I stirred the mixture and poured some into each of the tomato pots.

The tomatoes that grew after that all formed without the brown soft rot.

Do I have an education in horticulture? No. Have I taken one course? No. Like all of us, my education was not perfectly broad so I applied the knowledge I did have and used the Internet to expand what I knew into a very specific area.

What could Ben Franklin have accomplished if he had the Internet!

If a doctor can learn something useful about plants, a non-doctor can learn something about medicine - at least enough to work more effectively with your doctor.

One way to start to increase your understanding so you can ask pertinent questions is to look up online patient education materials. You need to avoid sites with bias. I'm suspicious of most of them that way.

Here's a good source of patient education material. Online is a marvelous medical reference website called **UpToDate.com**. Think of it as a 100,000-page textbook that gets updated every month as needed. You need to buy an expensive subscription for full access but the patient education materials are FREE. They come in "basic" and "beyond the basics" formats. Look up your topic in the search tab. Click the "patient" tab at the top.

See what is available. If they have something about your topic, that will take you to great articles. If you can't find anything under "acid in tomatoes" look up "ulcers."

I tried that for "peptic ulcer" which is the kind of ulcer you get from acid. The material does not mention tomatoes. If you read through the pH discussion you understand why. Tomatoes are not pertinent to peptic ulcers.

Don't be psyched out by what you don't know about medicine. All the knowledge of medicine is like a giant pizza. Think of a pizza with a ten-foot diameter. Like someone said about the song, "When the moon hits your eye like a big pizza pie," you'd better duck.

But if we slice that huge pizza into a few hundred slices, each slice is not complex. With a little study, a patient can learn a lot about one very narrow slice of the gigantic pizza which is the field of medicine.

You can figure out how many mushrooms and slices of pepperoni are on that one slice. You don't need to understand the whole pizza. It would be mind-boggling to analyze the entire ten-foot pizza, to know the total number of mushrooms and pepperoni bits. Just focus on that one slice first.

That is one reason why malpractice lawsuits are so frustrating to doctors. If a patient was harmed because the doctor forgot one single thing, an attorney can gather up and command a lot of knowledge after just a few hours of research. He/ she can command more knowledge about that one small slice of medicine than nine out of ten doctors.

If the malpractice attorney can do it, so can you. If my health depended on knowing something about that small slice of the medical pizza, I should find the time to get that information.

You don't use that knowledge to make life and death decisions about yourself. You use it to decide what to ask the doctor. You guide the discussion. You use it when you and your doctor discuss options.

Here is a situation. Your cardiologist refers you to a cardiac surgeon.

First visit: The surgeon says: "Sometime in the next year you need to have that leaky heart valve replaced. The operation takes a few hours and it will take about three months to fully recover from having your chest split open. Any questions? You are dumbfounded by the news and can't come up with any good questions.

After the visit you Google "aortic valve replacement options."

Within five minutes we find from The Mayo Clinic:

Aortic valve replacement surgery may be performed through traditional open-heart surgery or minimally invasive methods, which involve smaller incisions than those used in open-heart surgery.

Minimally invasive has an attractive ring to it, you think. You learn the recovery is a lot shorter with minimally invasive surgery. You learn that it is safer when done by surgeons with more experience in the new techniques.

At the next visit with the surgeon:

Patient: "Doctor, tell me about other options for replacing my valve, like with smaller incisions or other approaches. Don't they call that 'minimally invasive surgery?"

Surgeon: "We can do that. We have done that here."

You are not done asking questions:

"May I ask how many minimally-invasive valve replacements have you performed and what your mortality rate is after 30 days?"

That's pretty aggressive on your part, but it's your body, right? Maybe you just ask how many the surgeon has performed and wait on the morality rate question. If she/he says he has done only three minimally invasive cases you already know you want to check out other surgeons or medical centers.

You might feel you are just too timid to ask such bold questions of a doctor who is superbly trained, extremely hard working, and devoted to his/her patients. In that case, get a friend or relative to go with you. Someone like a retired nurse can help phrase bold questions in a respectful way.

If a patient comes to the doctor armed with some research, some ideas, and some thinking, the doctor might just listen.

No, please don't go to the doctor with 50 pages you printed out from the internet. Doctors don't want that. Chew on that information, digest what you can, do some reasoning, and then ask the doctor specific questions that matter to you.

Do Doctors Get Annoyed With Patients Who Save Up Ailments and Come With Four or Five Problems In One Appointment?

We are trained to not act annoyed. The most important issue to me in that situation was whether the four or five "problems" are all part of one disease process.

"I think I broke a bone in my foot," and "I have symptoms of a kidney stone," and "I'm drowsy and confused" are three separate conditions, right? No, they could all be symptoms of hyperparathyroidism, which causes elevated calcium, which, if high enough, can cause confusion, and leads to excess calcium elimination in the urine which in turn causes kidney stones and all the while the bones lose a bit of calcium every day from the elevated parathyroid levels and eventually stress fractures or worse can occur.

Having three connected symptoms is not the usual case. If the conditions are not connected, as a patient you have to ask yourself: "If the doctor has 15 minutes to spend with me and I give her/ him five different issues, that's three minutes for each one. If I came in with only one issue and the doctor spent only three minutes on my problem, would I trust him/her?"

Granted you don't need 15 minutes to look at a brown spot on the forearm.

Unfortunately for the better educated doctors, the higher the level of medical knowledge, the wider the range of possibilities that pop into the doctor's mind when he/she listens to you. Know less and the world of medicine becomes a simple place and you can get through your day faster. ☼

Have you noticed they want to call your doctor a "provider?" That's an "inclusive" term. You have already

258

noticed that more and more often the scheduler may offer you the physician assistant or the nurse practitioner? That will be OK if you have something routine. They might do a better job than a physician on a visit that is more routine. But when you have a new symptom and you see a practitioner with limited knowledge, your zebra won't be found.

See the chapter called "I am no genius," if you don't get the zebra reference.

If you have a new problem that does not seem routine and you see a doctor who won't spend the time to access all the knowledge in his/her brain or you see an "alternate provider" who won't bother the doctor she/he works with to get consultative diagnostic advice, you might just get that prescription promptly and be out of there on time. Hooray!!!

In a lot of offices if not most, the doctor is booked up and the nurse practitioner has openings. So if someone gets sick, they get to see the nurse practitioner. In my opinion, that's not just backwards, it's wrong.

As a physician, I could get frustrated that I would need to spend extra time with that patient who came in with five problems. Some issues would have to be deferred. But I needed to hear them all and decide which ones needed to be postponed.

These visits often went to twice the allowed time which annoyed some of my patients and always annoyed the office manager or so it seemed to me.

"Doctor, getting behind schedule will lower your satisfaction scores. The NP has higher satisfaction scores than you do, Doctor."

I had a chapter for this book on the topic of "Satisfaction Scores, a Tool of Satan." I was such a good chapter I had to remove it because it made the rest of the book look bad by comparison. ☺

If you are a doctor and you do listen to all the patient's concerns and pretend you are not in a hurry, someday a patient will disclose what she/he had that morning decided NOT to tell you. "Oh, by the way, I have another problem, which I haven't told anybody: I haven't been sleeping, I'm stressed out about life, and I'm thinking about whether I should kill myself."

A Patient Who Disclosed Thoughts of Suicide

"I'm thinking about whether I should kill myself." What does a doctor do if a patient says that?

During my training, I heard a lecture that I found disconcerting. A doctor explained how he managed a patient who revealed suicidal thoughts, not plans, at the end of an office visit. He said he quickly explained how much he cared and therefore wanted to see the patient next week when he could spend a full ten minutes on that problem!!!

Groan!

I must point out that patients sense the doctor doesn't have time for all their concerns. They see the doctor *standing* with his hand on the door knob. They tend to withhold some of their history when they see the doctor rushing through.

So dear prospective medical student: if you read this book and go into Family Medicine or Internal Medicine, I will notify you now that if you rush, the patient won't be as likely to bring up inconvenient matters like suicidal thoughts. That will help you stay on schedule and improve your satisfaction scores.

But be prepared. One day you may come to the office and your assistant will tell you, "You'll never guess what happened. That patient we saw last week committed suicide last night."

I am grateful that I never arrived at my office to be greeted by that kind of a shock.

What would I do when the patient hinted about suicide? I would ask questions about the patient's situation and address depression and suicidal ideation. Looking at my ruined schedule, I'd say to myself, "This is why I'm here. This is the most important visit of the day if not the week." If they had made *plans* to do the act or revealed other signs of being in danger, I would seek help from a psychiatrist that very day.

In my practice, I found a lot of patients who did not realize they were depressed. They presented with physical symptoms. The most common were fatigue, headache, GI symptoms, and backache.

When I explored for psychological symptoms most of them did not have sadness or crying among their complaints. To be clear some patients came in crying with a Kleenex box tucked under their arm and you did not need to be a detective to make the diagnosis. I am not saying everyone who is crying is depressed. I can hear Yoda's voice: "Different things they are - depression the mood and depression the illness."

When I probed for psychological symptoms, they commonly reported irritability, anxiety, difficulty focusing, thoughts that kept coming back over and over, and/or a sense of diminished self-esteem. One common symptom was anhedonia, the inability to enjoy life's pleasures: like a man who no longer enjoyed his hobbies. It was common for the patient to admit they were difficult to live with.

The irritability led to marital strain. Many times I thought that couples should not be allowed to divorce unless the possibility of depression had been explored and treated.

Most of these patients responded to antidepressants and cognitive counseling (examining with the patient their negative thoughts and how they affect their behavior and emotions) without seeing a psychiatrist.

I am hoping at least one reader of this book is inspired by understanding this chapter to save his/her life, or maybe even his/her marriage by getting treatment for this common disease. Bring up these thought if you have been having them. You can now call the suicide hot line or 988 in many parts of the country.

Kidneys: Yada Yada Yada

Jane Brody, the superb medical columnist for the NY Times, wrote about the encounter of a patient with Dr. Joseph Vassalotti in 2011.

The patient had early kidney failure. The kidney specialist had just offered a lengthy listing of what to do to prevent the future failure of the kidneys, so as to avoid the need for dialysis. The doctor stopped and asked, "What did I just say?" The patient replied, "Kidney disease: yada yada yada."

Naturally, there will be doctors who do more explaining and some who do less. But if you want to explain more, it's easy to lose the patient. In a lot of cases, the doctor is talking about something that quickly extends beyond the patient's field of experience. The patient is still thinking about the first two sentences and the physician is already on the fifth sentence. So we have to be very good at explaining. And after we explain by talking, we need to follow it up with the same information in writing.

How to best get the message across?

In Vaudeville, the performance was live. Unlike recorded TV or movies, live shows were performed repetitively, day after day, in city after city.

Today the method is to tape the scene or the skit. Do it again until the director is happy. Then edit the tapes, put them together into an episode, and next week record the next episode.

Maybe this difference is why Vaudeville was so successful. I once read that the best Vaudevillians depended on the response of the audience each night to improve their performance. Every night they tried doing their comedy routines a little differently, changed a word, or the timing, and then listened for the reaction of the audience. They did not have a director to please. They used the audience's laughter to gauge success. If a joke didn't get enough laughs one night, the good comic altered the delivery until it clicked. When the whole audience howled with laughter, the joke was set.

So that's the approach I tried for getting difficult messages across to my patients. I learned to watch the reaction of patients as I provided patient education. I used stories and corny analogies. When I could see the sparkle in the patient's eyes, I knew I was making contact. Then I would employ that way of explaining more often. I would also send the patient out with an educational "handout," whenever I had the chance.

263

But that did not mean the patient would retain the information. I might need to quiz the patient on the next visit to see what stuck and whether the patient had been able to follow the advice. If not, the next step was called, "Look for barriers." What got in the way?

The practice of medicine is paradoxical in a way. We invest a ton of research on finding the best diagnostic and treatment approaches. But how much do we spend on research showing the most effective way to convince patients to implement changes or to reduce risky practices?

One day I was trying to discuss with a doctor the best way to "sell" the patient on making beneficial changes. The doctor said, **"I don't sell 'em, I tell 'em."** I could see that would save a lot of time. This doctor had a reputation for staying on schedule and now that made perfect sense to me.

Maybe there should be professorships in the science of how to best educate and motivate patients. I recently returned to Princeton for my 50th reunion. When I was on campus I ran into a young woman who works in a new part of Princeton, the McGraw Center for Teaching and Learning which assesses and teaches University faculty how to better teach Princeton students. When I was at Princeton I had some brilliant teachers and some who were just brilliant in their fields but not so much in teaching. I wish this innovation would spread to our healthcare system. After all, the word "doctor" derives from the Latin "docere" which means "to teach."

For People With Early Kidney Disease: A Guide re What Can You Do To Prevent The Advance of Kidney Failure?

I couldn't tell the yada yada story without providing the list of what to do if you have early kidney disease:

a. Aggressively control blood pressure. Keep the systolic under 130 and the diastolic under 80.

b. Aggressively control diabetes. For every drop of A1c of 1%, the risk of renal failure drops by 40%.

c. Lose weight – very important.

d. Drink enough fluids to avoid kidney stones but avoid excessive colas.

e. Limit protein in the diet. Take enough but not too much. Your doctor can advise you on how much. Some Americans take far more protein than is needed and that taxes the kidneys. The recommended amount is 0.36 grams of protein per pound of weight. For the average man, it's 56 grams, for the average woman, 43 grams per day. To figure your protein intake, you have to write down what you eat, study the food labels, and do some math.

f. Avoid excess sodium and potassium. Your doctor can check if your potassium is creeping up which can become dangerous if too high.

g. Avoid drugs that harm the kidneys: NSAIDS (Aspirin, Advil, Naprosyn, etc). Check with your doctor. Some patients will get away with an occasional dose of these drugs if the kidney disease is truly early. Daily usage is much more of a problem. Discuss with your physician.

h. Avoid high-dose x-ray dye (remind your doctor to be careful when you have a test that needs dye injected).

i. If you start a statin for cholesterol, let your doctor know when you first take if you get severe muscle pain. That could signify a release of muscle enzymes that can harm the kidneys. The clue for that release of enzymes would be the severe muscle pain. That is uncommon.

j. Avoid laxatives and antacids that contain magnesium and aluminum (Mylanta and Milk of Magnesia).

k. Avoid ulcer drugs like Tagamet and Zantac and Pepcid but especially avoid reflux drugs like Nexium and Prilosec can also cause kidney damage.

l. Decongestants like Sudafed can harm the kidneys. Read labels carefully. Some cold products contain both decongestants and Ibuprofen.

m. Avoid enemas that contain phosphorus (Fleet).

n. Avoid Aka-Seltzer, which is high in salt. Avoid: sodium bicarbonate as a stomach remedy, same reason.

o. Whether supplements harm the kidneys is often difficult to look up. Beware of supplements. Be very cautious.

p. At every visit ask your doctor to review your medications concerning prevention of harm to the kidneys.

"The Child is Father of the Man" What Does That Actually Mean?

My heart leaps up when I behold
A rainbow in the sky:
So was it when my life began;
So is it now I am a man;
So be it when I shall grow old,
Or let me die!
The Child is father of the Man;
And I could wish my days to be
Bound each to each by natural piety.

William Wordsworth wrote that in 1802.

I did not understand this "the child is father" paradox when I was in college.

I was always struck by the unfairness of childhood. Habits and decisions you make in your junior high school and high school years can control your future. Did you force yourself to be disciplined? Did you teach yourself to listen in school?

Do you make it a practice to consider options or do you act impulsively? Can you adequately evaluate the risk versus benefit of your decisions, such as whether to speed when driving, whether to do drugs or expose yourself to sexually transmitted diseases?

Try becoming a doctor (or similar professions that require extensive training) if you have not developed good study skills by the end of junior high school. It's possible but it wouldn't be easy or likely. How unfair it is that a person fails to achieve medical school admission due to bad decisions at age 12?

When I applied to medical school there were 2.2 premed college applicants for every one who got accepted to at least one school. At a particular medical school, it might have been only one in ten accepted. In 2019 it was 2.4 applicants for every one who got in overall.

Each future doctor still needs every asset he or she had developed.

Where did that mature 8th grader come from? The 8th grader produced herself from the 6th grader she had been 2 years earlier.

From where did the 6th grader arise? From the elementary school pupil.

Where did that elementary school child get his nature and habits? From the parents and genes.

So the parents give birth to the young child and form that child until a certain age when the child learns to either accept or reject traits that will form his/her future character.

The child has a big role in deciding which way to go. The strength of the influence of the parents' verbal teaching wanes but the influence of the parents' example is much more powerful.

I attribute the success of my four children to my wife. She was with them for so many more hours than I was. Yes, I had some time to help with their homework and we did all kinds of things together.

I would come home from my medical office at 7 PM, or 8 PM or even later. What were the kids doing when I came home? They were working on their homework. Their long hours matched mine. If I'd been out bowling and drinking beer with friends, would they have developed their work ethic?

Albert Schweitzer famously wrote: "Example is not the main thing in influencing others; it is the only thing."

I recall the story of the frustrated mother of a teenage daughter. The mother had made bad decisions as a teenager resulting in her becoming an unwed mother, estrangement from her parents, economic deprivation, poor choices in men, use of intoxicants, etc.

Now she says, "I can't believe it. I told my daughter exactly what to do to have a better life and she wound up making the same mistakes I made."

A Random and Unplanned Life-changing Event

It was definitely a random and unplanned life-changing event. I was nine and our family had just joined a swim pool that had opened for its first season. One morning, the kid three doors down on our street told me he was trying out for the swim team later that day, so I went too. I swam 25 meters in 30 seconds. That was pretty slow compared to the other kids. I recall having difficulty with my right arm recovery. I didn't have the shoulder flexibility to recover on top of the water so it was kind of a "drag your arm forward under the water" recovery on that arm, if you can picture that.

The next day, I figured out how to fix the problem and in the first meet I did the 25 meters in 21 seconds. In two weeks I went from one of the slowest to the fastest in my age group. This was the pool's first season so every time I had a best time, it was a club record. My sister also swam with the team and became the best in her age group. Pretty soon swimming was our favorite family activity.

I figured out that some swimmers were faster because they had better technique. I studied the strokes of the faster swimmers. I asked the coaches for advice. We had one girl on the team who was very good, that first year I swam. I recall she was about 16 which to me, as a nine-year old, was quite a mature age. The two coaches were helping me learn better swim technique by having me watch this girl swim back and forth in the diving well. From the vantage of the pool deck, I could see how she swam on top but I wondered how she pulled her arms under the water. In 1959 they didn't show underwater shots on TV and of course, there was no YouTube to teach yourself things.

In those days only skin and scuba divers wore goggles. I said to the coaches, both men, that if I could get some

269

goggles, I would like to dive below her as she swam and "study her form." The coaches thought this was hilarious. I could not understand why they thought it was so funny. I made a mental footnote and figured I'd probably understand it when I was older.

Before that summer, I had never considered myself an athlete. I couldn't do any sport particularly well. I remember learning the word "athlete" earlier that year and saying to myself, "I'm not that." But that summer I guess I became an athlete.

At the end of the summer some of the football players of my age, having learned of my accomplishments in the pool, came to my home and asked if I wanted to try out for a football team. I said, "No thanks, I'm a swimmer." After that, I swam every winter and summer.

At age 12, I won five individual state championship gold medals in New Jersey. I was hooked.

I entered a slump for two years after that. I couldn't achieve the times I had when I was 12. I guess I didn't know how to use the new body I was developing. But I just stuck with it.

At age 15, I dropped times like crazy. My 100-yard freestyle time fell from 58.5 at age 14 to 50.8 at 15. That year the NCAA men's swimming champion for the 100-yard freestyle won in 46.1. I was only 4.7 seconds slower. That time by a 15-year-old got the attention of Princeton's swim coach, Olympic Gold Medalist Bob Clotworthy. He wrote me a lot of letters. During my senior year I chose Princeton over Harvard, which I never regretted.

A decade after I started swimming I was representing Princeton at the NCAA Championships. I was an average swimmer at that level of competition. I earned an All-American certificate for a relay when I was 19.

In my senior year, I applied to just one medical school. In 1970 that was a big mistake. Only 45% of pre-med students were accepted into any medical school in those days. The odds of getting into your first choice were even lower. Most college students in my situation applied to many, many places. But I wanted to go to Cincinnati. My Dad had died when I was in high school and my mother lived alone in the Cincinnati area. I'd been away for four years. It was time to be closer to home.

It was Thanksgiving weekend of my senior year and I was 21. I had driven my motorcycle 660 miles from Princeton, New Jersey to Cincinnati in the rain. That was a very cold and wet trip. I was interviewing with the Dean of the Medical School. Over his shoulder, I could see the building across the street, and the window of the corner hospital room where my father had died four years earlier.

It was the etiquette of these interviews that you should not ask if you were going to get accepted. I was anxious on that score, to be sure. I told the dean something like this, "My mother is a widow and she lives here. That's why I decided Cincinnati would be the only school to which I would apply. Do you think applying to one school was a mistake?"

The dean said something like: "Well, Bob, I am looking at your record and can see you got good grades. But nearly all our applicants have grades like yours. I see you were on the swimming team for all four years. That tells me you have what you need to do the work at this school. I would say you are definitely going to get into at least one medical school."

A month later I received a letter. I was accepted. I actually swam into medical school.

After college graduation, I returned to Cincinnati. Medical school was a very busy time. I quit swimming. Big mistake. For 22 years, I got way out of shape.

By age 43, I had three kids on the Y swim team. I thought exercise was walking down an 80-foot driveway to the mailbox. Lucky for me, the Y had two pools, so in time I started swimming in one pool, while the kids would be practicing with their team in the other. I gradually got back into shape.

Then I heard about Masters Swimming. My wife was explaining it to her sister who didn't understand it at first. Finally she said, "Oh, I get it...swim meets for old farts!"

I went to the meets for old farts.

Our team had a motto: "The older we get, the faster we were." Eventually I had medaled at several Masters' National Swim Championship meets. I had a dozen or more Top 10 USA rankings in my age group, usually 10th. There is a saying in Masters Swimming: "Top 10 before topsoil." In 2000, at the Masters' World Championship in Germany, I earned a sixth-place medal in my age group in the 200 meter freestyle. That was the highlight of my Masters Swimming career.

I haven't quit swimming since that time. I used to practice because I had a meet coming up but now I just swim. I stopped competing over a decade ago. I swim about 20 miles a month just for the exercise. As I get older, I swim slower and don't worry about it.

Going to that swim team tryout when I was nine changed my life.

Sometimes I share a lane with a younger swimmers. I hope swimming will do as much for them as it did for me. I tell them, "Once I swam in a meet and touched the finish before Michael Phelps."

"No way!" they say. "How'd you do that?"

I answer, "He hadn't been born yet."

You can say this if you have been swimming long enough.

Family History Young vs Old Relations

A lot of people don't know this concept.

If some medical condition runs in the family and showed up when your ancestors were young, the condition would more likely be genetic. ☼

If it happened when your relatives were older people, it's more likely related to age and environment or your relative's health habits. That family history would be less of a worry for you.

So if your brother had a heart attack at the young age of 41, you might get on cholesterol medication even if your cholesterol looks good. You might start an exercise program. You might be motivated to really watch that waist measurement (as in the essay on insulin resistance.)

But if your grandfather died of a heart attack at age 90 there is less to worry about. You might even find it reassuring that his heart disease had advanced so slowly that it took 90 years to kill him.

Thinking Errors

To be a patient who participates in decision-making and doesn't want to be harmed by his/her medical care, you need to know that your doctor, like all of us, may be subject to "THINKING ERRORS."

We don't always think right. We all make errors. Not just all doctors, but all people.

Once I was drawing blood from a patient with poor veins. I knew those veins well. I always had good luck with one vein which came close to the surface at just one spot on the arm. As I pulled out the needle I realized I had forgotten I needed another tube of a different color.

I told her I was sorry but I had just made a mistake.

She looked totally shocked.

When I recognized what her face was saying I asked, "Didn't you know I could make a mistake?" She had a one-word response, "No."

Doctors all make mistakes.

Get over it. What should matter to patients would be whether they were found before they caused harm.

I am going to explain a type of thinking error called the Monte Carlo fallacy. This error is an underlying mental error in the psychology of gambling. It seems intuitive when flipping a coin that following a series of ten heads in a row, it is much more likely that the next coin flip will be tails. That is an erroneous but common belief. Those who have studied probability know that the chance of tails at the next coin flip is 50-50. Even if just before that you had ten heads in a row, the odds of tails are 50% each time.

Note: in this book the chance of tales is 100%.

Under the Monte Carlo fallacy, a slot machine that has not had a winner for a while is thought more likely to have a winner before the other slot machines.

The Monte Carlo fallacy just doesn't make sense with slot machines unless there is some electrical network from each slot to the master computer that controls these things. Otherwise, there is no secret device that tells the one machine it's time for it to pay a jackpot or not.

Similarly, under the "hot-hand fallacy" the gaming table is not "hot." Just because there have been a string of winners, it's NOT likely to have more winners tonight than the usual odds would predict. The odds always predict that the house will win on average.

Doctors are also subject to the belief that events can happen in streaks when in reality they are separate and random. ☼

Let's say a doctor has the following unfortunate experience. He/she sees a patient with an innocent-sounding cough. That is usually bronchitis. The cough is treated in the usual way. Two months later, the patient comes back. The cough has persisted. A chest x-ray seems like a good idea. Unfortunately, lung cancer is discovered. Invariably, that doctor may start ordering a lot more chest x-rays when other patients come in with a cough. If the doctor is hit with a malpractice suit over this point, the extra chest x-rays are even more likely.

I want to point out that if researchers ever determine that detecting lung cancer two months earlier makes a difference, we will get a chest x-ray for many more patients with cough on the first visit.

Similarly when a doctor ignores a one in 100 possibility, of something that would be a disaster not to find, and gets away with ignoring it ten times in a row, he/she learns incorrectly that he/she doesn't have to consider that possibility. If you have seen 100 sick kids with viruses and never saw a case of meningitis, you cannot "learn" from that streak that you don't need to consider meningitis with a sick child. You still have to carefully look for and work up the sick kids that show the warning signs of meningitis.

The hot-hand fallacy and the Monte Carlo fallacy also affect the decision-making of patients.

Say you find out that two friends came down with breast cancer. You decide to get a mammogram earlier than the guidelines recommend. Those cancers were chance events. You are not more likely to get breast cancer because your two friends did. Just do what is recommended, on the recommended schedule, not more often.

A woman wanted to get a Pap smear early because her sister just learned she had cancer of the cervix. But cancer of the cervix is transmitted by virus and has nothing to do with genetics or family history. So get the pap every three to five years as recommended, not earlier than that because twenty years ago your sister had caught the virus that gave her cancer of the cervix now. You don't inherit cancer of the cervix. It's sexually transmitted from HPV (virus).

Another point: getting a mammogram every year instead of every two years has been shown to greatly increase the rate of false alarms without helping. Unless you are behind the normal screening schedule, don't get a mammogram just because your friend got breast cancer.

Another thinking error is a type of bias known as the availability heuristic or familiarity bias. In 1994 Lucian Leape of the Harvard School of Public Health called out this error, the tendency for the practitioner to use the first idea that comes to mind. If a doctor had just gone to a lecture about an uncommon disease or had seen a patient with that condition, she/he is more likely to test for that disease for weeks or even months afterward.

Or if a doctor just sat through a promotional presentation about a new drug, he/she is more likely to order that drug because it becomes "available" when it pops into the doctor's mind. When he/she lifts his pen (or mouse) to choose what to prescribe, the thought of that drug comes to mind even if the physician did not like the presentation or disagreed with parts of it.

The entire philosophy behind advertising depends on this thinking error, the availability heuristic.

When your doctor tests you for a rare disease, is that a sound idea or is it just the result of having just attended a lecture on that topic?

Leape described many other types of errors of medical thinking. Some are simply the result of time pressure or fatigue or stress or being distracted or reliance on memory. The error called "reliance on memory" acknowledges that our memories are always imperfect. Computers can help us overcome this weakness by showing us lists or checklists.

Latent errors are those set up by poor system design and are known as "accidents waiting to happen." Think of similar-sounding drug names or two patients on the same floor with the same last name.

Decision-making by rules known as guidelines, generally helps reduce error but sometimes the wrong rule is applied. The guideline the doctor remembers is for patients aged 50 to 70. The patient is 75. That causes the error. Another guideline calls for three different approaches based on the status of the patient. The doctor lumps all three together when he memorizes the guideline.

Reliance on memory contributes to many errors.

Since we are all susceptible to a whole range of fallacious thinking or thinking errors, it helps to have the patient and the physician thinking together to achieve a logical approach to decision making. ☼ "Informed consent" is now the law of the land. But sometimes the "informing" is not performed as well as it should be to catch thinking errors by the doctor or by the patient.

Occam's Razor: the Less Complex Possibility is More Likely to be Right

The wiser patient knows a bit about how doctors think. Occam's Razor is a principle in problem-solving employed by scientists and doctors. It is attributed to an English friar and philosopher, William of Ockham who died in 1347. The idea is that when there are two competing explanations or theories for a phenomenon, the simpler one is more likely true. ☼ Each potential explanation, theory, or diagnosis contains a number of assumptions. The more complex alternative contains either more assumptions or more elaborate assumptions and is more likely to be wrong.

A phenomenon: the food in the oven was burned.

One possibility, the simple one: it was cooked too long.

A alternate possibility, more complex: when the cook wasn't looking someone turned up the oven temperature from 375 to 450 for 30 minutes and then turned it back down just before the timer buzzed.

We should consider Occam's Razor when deciding on a diagnosis when there are several possibilities.

When the patient has five symptoms, the doctor needs to search for a single cause that might explain all the symptoms.

Let's say the patient has (1) heartburn, (2) weight loss, (3) chest pain, (4) exacerbation of asthma, and (5) cough.

This would be the approach of the doctor not employing Occam's Razor:

(1) Heartburn is due to excess acid. That gets treated with an acid blocker,

(2) The weight loss could be due to cancer: order CT scan of the abdomen plus upper and lower endoscopies.

(3) The chest pain could be the heart: order a treadmill test and a cardiology consult.

(4) The asthma could be getting worse because of pollen or a virus which are the most common reasons. Send the patient to the allergist.

(5) The cough could be due to pneumonia, order a chest x-ray.

In contrast, this could be the thinking of the doctor employing Occam's razor:

(1)Listen carefully.

(2) Pursue other related symptoms.

(3) Think of options before deciding what tests to order, and what medicine to prescribe.

(4) Are there other possibilities besides the first one I thought of? Can I think of a single condition that explains several of the symptoms?

Analysis: The heartburn could be due to the reflux of acid into the lower esophagus. It usually is. The discomfort interferes with eating. Could that be why the patient has lost weight? The inflamed esophagus could be causing the pain in the chest. Ask if it's worse to lie down. Some of the acid gets up way beyond the lower esophagus. The high refluxing acid goes all the way up to the larynx. The stream of air during inspiration picks up tiny droplets of that acid-containing stomach fluid. The droplets are inhaled into the lungs setting off an exacerbation of the patient's pre-existing asthma. The cough is likely due to the asthma exacerbation and not a separate lung problem such as pneumonia.

Hypothesis: all five symptoms are related to acid reflux.

Plan: quiz the patient more carefully about the chest pain. Pain from reflux would not be related to exertion so that issue needs to be clarified.

Consider the patient's other cardiac risk factors (age, smoking, cholesterol, family history, exercise habit, presence of hypertension.) If it does not sound like it could be cardiac pain, the treatment is to reduce the acid with a Proton Pump Inhibitor, PPI, such as omeprazole, and bring the patient back in two weeks to see if the other five symptoms have improved. If symptoms sound like they could be cardiac, then proceed with a cardiac workup because Occam's Razor, telling us there is a single, simple explanation, is not always right.

Quiz: for the reader who remembers a recent chapter.

Five symptoms:

Headache. Backache. Fatigue. GI upset. Trouble sleeping.

Ideas?

Not using Occam's Razor: Treat the headache, backache and GI distress with separate medications and prescribe a sleeping pill for the sleeping problem.

Using Occam's Razor: Evaluate for depression. Avoid the sleeping pill, they are "downers," and could worsen depression. Explain to the patient what you are thinking. Start an antidepressant. In two weeks see if the patient is beginning to feel better.

Waiting, Waiting, My Doctor's Kept Me Waiting

The last time my doctor kept me waiting 45 minutes I said, "Thank you for being the kind of doctor who will spend extra time with patients, when needed. Also I got to read four chapters in the book I brought with me."

Optimism

I was inspired listening to George Takei on NPR. George once said, "I was going to start a club for pessimists but I was afraid it wouldn't work."

George also said something like this, "PESSIMISTS ARE DEFEATED FROM THE START. ALL HUMAN PROGRESS COMES FROM OPTIMISTS." ☼

I know this concept is oversimplified. All of us have a mixture of both optimism and pessimism in our makeup. But I think the only advantage of being consistently pessimistic is the certainty you won't be disappointed. You won't fail at something you care about.

How's that? If you believe you will never succeed in fixing a problem, you are certain not to fail because you will never have tried anything. You have to try in order to fail. No failures for you!

When working with doctors who made errors, I used to counsel them: "The only people who never make mistakes are the ones who never do anything."

I also read that all dogs are optimists. Maybe that's why we like them so much. How do we know dogs are optimists? To chase after a car, with no idea what you're going to do once you catch up, you have to be an optimist. Just think about it.

That joke makes a point. Simply throwing caution to the winds and believing in your success is not what I mean. That kind of naïveté can produce the most profound type of stupid acts. That dog doesn't consider the consequences were he ever to catch that speeding car. You don't have to try out every idea if you know it's risky.

No, what I mean by optimism is an underlying belief that a successful, reasonable, and safe solution to the problem is discoverable, *eventually*.

In other words, it is a practical approach to problem-solving to assume you will eventually find a solution to the problem at hand.

Some medical conditions are tough to diagnose or treat. When the patient has tried the local specialists, then traveled to a major medical center and then at a national medical center such as The Mayo Clinic or the Cleveland Clinic, the optimistic patient comes back to the family doctor. We try something else and then something else and sometimes we find something that works. Optimism is important for the success of both the patient and the doctor. ☼ Keep trying.

"Nothing in this world can take the place of persistence. Talent will not; nothing is more common than unsuccessful men with talent. Genius will not; unrewarded genius is almost a proverb. Education will not; the world is full of educated derelicts. Persistence and determination alone are omnipotent. The slogan 'Press On!' has solved and always will solve the problems of the human race." Calvin Coolidge

Prevention of Large Artery Arterial Disease (Strokes and Heart Attacks) Part I: The Things You Cannot Alter

Heart disease is the leading cause of death. *Yawn. Heard that already.* Heart disease kills 635,000 Americans per year. *Yawn, most of them are just old, right?* Heart disease causes 23% of all deaths. *Yawn, another statistic Gotta die from something.*

Then suddenly, somebody you know dies of heart disease: a grandparent, a former teacher, your friend's mom, your college roommate, whoever. *Hey maybe heart disease is something I need to know more about.*

We call it Cardiovascular Disease. Cardio means heart and vascular means blood vessel.

There are no secrets hidden behind some curtain, for the most part. Those who read up learn that most of what is called cardiovascular disease is caused by vascular disease, disease in the arteries. You may have heard of it as "blocked arteries."

By the way, when the doctor says the artery is blocked, a lot of patients think it's 100% blocked. Like a roadblock. But doctors use "blocked" or "obstructed" in reference to partial obstructions. "The Circumflex coronary artery had a 50% obstruction three centimeters from the origin."

One more thing: a 50% obstruction or narrowing does not reduce the flow by that much. Up to a point, the blood just goes faster through the narrow part.

We know how to reduce the risk of blocked arteries. Sometimes I think that your doctor has gone over this stuff with so many patients that he/ she believes that everybody knows this. ☼

I am going to present eight cardiac risk factors. In my experience, most people cannot recall all eight.

A moment of clarity is in order. One goal in life should be to avoid or delay nasty diseases like heart attack or stroke. I'd also like to avoid being struck by a lightning bolt or being eaten by a shark which are very uncommon ways of going to your maker. Stroke and heart attack are much more common and very much worth studying how to avoid.

A little anatomy if you are new to all this: from the heart the oxygen-rich blood travels out through arteries. Larger ones branch off to smaller ones called arterioles and they in turn lead to the smallest vessels called capillaries.

Only through these tiny capillaries does the work get done. Oxygen and nutrients leave the red blood cells for the tissues. Carbon dioxide, the byproduct of oxidative metabolism, is taken up by the red blood cells in the capillaries. These tiny capillaries then combine to form venules or little veins, which combine to form larger veins.

A point to understand is that the body has a plethora of veins, a lot of redundancy. You can lose many veins and still live. But large arteries are not as numerous. In many cases, a highly blocked artery leads to a big problem in the territory downstream that the artery was supposed to supply with fresh oxygen and nutrients. Examples: heart attack and stroke.

The arteries that supply fresh blood to the heart muscle are called the coronary arteries. The ones that feed the brain are cerebral arteries. If the blood flow gets seriously slowed down or even shut down, the tissues downstream can die.

These arteries can gradually get blocked by plaque composed of cholesterol and proteins, or they can be blocked suddenly by a clot. Often the clot forms at the site of the plaque, especially if the plaque is new or inflamed.

It's important to understand this, so here's a quiz.

Match the letter and the number

A: Blocked Coronary Artery   1: Stroke

B: Blocked Cerebral Artery   2: Heart Attack

C: Sudden Blockage   3:Cholesterol plaque

D: Gradual Blockage   4: Clot forming on a plaque

Answer: A2, B1, C4, D3

If you passed the quiz, you can move on.

What can we do to prevent these arteries from becoming blocked up? We identify what we call *risk factors* and then work on each one of them.

The problems that predict large artery disease fall into two categories: Fixed risk factors which cannot be changed. And alterable risk factors, just the opposite. When you improve or eliminate these risk factors, you might reduce the risk.

I said I can list eight factors that control your risk for the type of large artery arterial disease that leads to heart attack and stroke. I will mention that disease of the smaller arteries can be important but small artery disease is less well understood and is less common except in people with diabetes.

We count three FIXED risk factors for large artery arteriosclerotic diseases (heart attack and stroke). We call them "fixed" because these three cannot be altered. You cannot do anything about your sex, your age, or your family history.

Number one: Your sex: You cannot change it, at least genetically. Here's the fact to memorize: Men tend to get their arterial disease about 10 years earlier than women with everything else being equal. ☼

Number two is age. Age is the strongest risk factor. Age is a killer. Even when all the other risk factors are good, as you get older, the risk of large vessel arterial disease climbs sharply. You cannot stop aging. Birthdays are bad for you, but you can't have a long life without a lot of them.

In Through the Looking Glass (Lewis Carroll) Alice said "One can't help growing older"

'So here's a question for you. How old did you say you were?'

Alice made a short calculation, and said 'Seven years and six months.'

'Wrong!' Humpty Dumpty exclaimed triumphantly. 'You never said a word like it!'

'I thought you meant "How old **are** you?"' Alice explained.

'If I'd meant that, I'd have said it,' said Humpty Dumpty.

Alice didn't want to begin another argument, so she said nothing.

'Seven years and six months!' Humpty Dumpty repeated thoughtfully. 'An uncomfortable sort of age. Now if you'd asked **my** advice, I'd have said "Leave off at seven" — but it's too late now.'

'I never ask advice about growing,' Alice said indignantly.

'Too proud?' the other enquired.

Alice felt even more indignant at this suggestion. 'I mean,' she said, 'that one can't help growing older.'

Let's just say that the only sure way to avoid dying from the effects of old age is to die young from something else. I don't recommend that.

Number three: The third fixed risk factor for large vessel cardiovascular disease is family history.

It is a strong risk factor if you have a history of heart attack in younger relatives specifically men under the age of 56 and women under the age of 66. A heart attack in a 90-year-old father or grandfather is not so suspicious to a physician. ☼

Many people have wanted to do so, but you cannot lose your relatives. You can't change your family history. You can understand it better by knowing how old people were when they developed their diseases.

One of my favorite parts in Oscar Wilde's "The Importance of Being Earnest:"

Lady Bracknell: Are your parents living?

Jack Worthing: I have lost both my parents.

Lady Bracknell: To lose one parent, Mr. Worthing, may be regarded as a misfortune; to lose both looks like carelessness.

People with a cardiac family history need to be aggressive about the other arterial risk factors.

Prevention of Large Artery Arterial Disease (Strokes and Heart Attacks) Part II: The Things You Can Alter

Before getting to these five alterable risk factors, a little more anatomy is needed. Recall that the arteries carry blood to all parts of the body. The veins bring the blood back to the heart and lungs.

The arteries have three layers. The outer layer is tough and that makes it useful for surgeons when they sew the artery when doing a bypass operation. The middle layer is muscular and allows arteries to dilate and constrict. The inner layer is called the intima, a word that sounds like "intimate."

Intimate sleepwear is very thin and nearly transparent. It's not for cold nights in the northern climates. The arterial intima is likewise very thin but it is critical to the function of the artery. Cholesterol deposits that block up arteries are formed between the intima and the muscular layer.

During the Korean War, the U.S. Army started doing autopsies on soldiers who died in battle. The pathologists discovered that men in their 20s were already starting to get deposits of cholesterol in the space between the intima and the middle muscular layer.

That accumulation of cholesterol debris is called plaque. Doctors realized in the 1950s that arteriosclerosis is a lifelong process, not just something that begins in older people.☼

We used to think what happened was something like this: the plaque grew progressively year after year, the usable inside diameter of the artery became smaller and smaller with the plaque gradually blocking the flow through the artery. Finally it closed off the artery. "Bingo!" that's a heart attack or a stroke.

That concept has been replaced by a better idea: a clot could form suddenly on a damaged section of plaque.

Why would a clot form right in the middle of an important heart artery or brain artery? The thinking is that sometimes the intima is split by something. It gets a little crack or a fissure. Or perhaps it develops some inflammation which attracts clot.

Imagine a very well-built garden hose with three layers. The inner layer is flexible rubber. The middle layer is a steel mesh. The outer layer is shiny plastic. The split happens in the inner rubber layer.

Platelets are floating past the split. These platelets are tiny, about 50,000 of them in a cubic millimeter of blood. They don't have brains of their own; they work automatically reacting to their environment. If they had a simple brain and eyes they might look at the crack in the intimal layer and say, "Look at that! That looks a lot like a little shaving cut. Come on guys, we'd better stop here and close it up." At that point thousands of little platelets would stick together and form a clot at the site of the intimal tear. They have no clue it's not a shaving cut. They have no clue it's the inside of your brain or heart artery and they have no clue that clots are big trouble there.

So one way of keeping yourself from arterial diseases is to consider: "How do I take good care of my arteries' intimal layer?" ☼ Can you imagine your doctor asking, "How's your intima?"

With the anatomy in mind, here are the five correctible risk factors.

******************** 1 ******************

Lack of adequate aerobic exercise: thought to be responsible for 9% of all premature deaths. We tend to recommend 30 minutes, five times a week or 150 minutes per week. You don't have to exhaust yourself to get something out of it, but driving around the golf course in a golf cart probably doesn't hack it. Sorry golfers who use carts. When you exercise hard enough and long enough the arteries, including the coronary arteries, dilate throughout the body. You don't want to go for weeks and weeks and weeks without having your coronary arteries dilate. Work that intima!

******************** 2 ******************

Lack of control of the blood pressure: probably the first thing most people think of but it's is the least important of the five correctible risk factors. More people are working on this risk factor than the other four. When needed, add medication to keep the systolic average under 140. Losing weight often does the trick. Avoiding excessive sodium might work or help at least.

******************** 3 ******************

Not being on a statin when your cholesterol indicates high risk. It's traditional to call this risk factor hyperlipidemia or hypercholesterolemia or elevated LDL cholesterol. Why stress statins? Treating cholesterol with drugs that are not statins seems to have a minimal effect on the rate of heart attack and stroke compared to the results with statins.

High risk: high cholesterol.

Lower risk: being on a statin.

Plain English: all the drugs other than statins barely work if at all. Look at Repatha (evolocumab) the new $6000 per year cholesterol drug.

They sell it for lowering LDL when you are not getting to goal on a statin alone.

Where's the evidence about reducing heart attack and stroke with Repatha? Here is the first paragraph of the abstract from the May 2017 article in the New England Journal of Medicine:

"Evolocumab is a monoclonal antibody that inhibits proprotein convertase subtilisin–kexin type 9 (PCSK9) and lowers low-density lipoprotein (LDL) cholesterol levels by approximately 60%. Whether it prevents cardiovascular events is uncertain."

Well, that was a key sentence, that last one. Spend $6000 a year to improve your lab tests. Then a study came out that followed 27,000 patients for two years and found that 5.9% of high-risk patients who combined Repatha with a statin suffered a heart attack, stroke, or died, compared with 7.4% of patients who took a statin plus a placebo. According to a research letter to the editor of JAMA, this works out to one patient helped for 37 treated for a cost per year of quality life gained of $450,000. That's the cost of adding one year of life. Naturally, insurance companies have been reluctant to cover this drug.

Note that this was a test of the Repatha PLUS a statin. I think we have to spend most of our efforts getting people on a statin first.

That's why I'm calling this third risk factor "Not being on a statin." As you get older your cholesterol might look pretty good as far as fitting within normal values. But what does *normal* really do for you? Normal values are defined as the range where 90% of patients values fall. *Normal* means "like most everyone else" but it does not necessarily mean "good" for you.☼ Yet even when cholesterol is *normal*, the risk of heart attack and stroke can be high due to that nasty fixed risk factor age. There are a lot of older patients with "*normal*" cholesterol but unacceptably high cholesterol risk numbers. In that case, statins will still reduce the risk enough to be worthwhile. If your ten year risk of a heart attack or stroke over the next ten years calculates to 15%, statins might drop it to 10%. That an NNT of 20. Treat 20 people, save one heart attack or stroke. Statins are not expensive and if they don't cause you side effects, why not?

One further distinction. Preventing a heart attack in someone who never has been known to have coronary artery disease and has no symptoms is called Primary Prevention. The NNT (number needed to treat before one patient is helped) with statins is higher in the primary prevention group. Trying to prevent a heart attack by prescribing a statin to someone who is known to have coronary heart disease is more productive. The NNT is lower.

That makes sense if you think about it. Statins are likely to help those with high risk. By analogy, if you could install something in a car to prevent speeding, that device might save a bunch of lives. But if you had only a limited number of those speed-control devices, you'd install them in the cars of teenagers. That's where you'd get the best bang for the buck. Most people on the older end of the age spectrum have learned to slow down and stay close to the speed limit. For most trips around town, people who follow the speed limit arrive at their destination only a minute or two later. ☼

I was thinking about adding that statins were not recommended after the age of 75 due to lack of evidence. But...I double checked that and found that a 2020 study of 327,000 veterans 75 and older showed a 25% reduction in all-cause death and a 20% reduction in heart disease-related death for statin users with no heart disease.

Some people develop side effects on statins and can't take them. But about half the people who are reasonably sure they can't take statins find on the second try that they don't have side effects after all.

Lots of people knock statins. It seems like the more popular and successful a medication, the more people will make up lies or repeat incorrect ideas about its harmful effects.

For example, Prozac is the most successful medication for depression and yet it is the psychoactive drug that people are most fearful of for no good reason.

Immunizations are magnificently successful so what do the fear mongers focus on: immunizations. Likewise, statins are in the crosshairs of these medically ignorant people.

How do statins help protect the intima layer? They probably stabilize or harden the inner layer so that it doesn't split. This effect is based on the reduction of inflammation in the inner lining.

This next point is amazing. Someone did a dental study on statins and found that the patients taking statins had less gum inflammation. That was pretty interesting because gum inflammation has been correlated with heart attack risk. Yes, if you don't take good care of your gums, the risk of heart attack goes up. So it's possible that flossing your teeth may help your heart. And statins may help your gums. But up to now, we don't include gum disease with the major risk factors for arterial disease. But maybe I should have called this risk factor "Not taking a statin for high risk and not flossing your teeth."

*********************4*******************

The fourth correctible risk factor for large artery disease is **hyperinsulinism** or insulin resistance or we could call it

292

the big waist. The official teachings on this subject will split this risk factor into three things (a) obesity, (b) diabetes, and (c) poor diet. Often cited under poor diet is the lack of fruit and vegetables. I think once you understand the effect of high insulin levels on the coronary arteries, you understand these three are all related.

That's why I lump them together.

But even listing all three does not give the whole story. It's not just obesity. Even being overweight, the category below obese and above normal, will result in insulin resistance if the excess fat is around the middle, which is where it usually is. Insulin resistance causes extra insulin production. **High Insulin levels give rise to arterial plaque**.

When you have insulin resistance your pancreas needs to make more insulin which it does until it can't keep up with the high demand. Then you cross over into diabetes. But you have increased coronary artery risk with pre-diabetes too, so we need to be listing *diabetes* and *pre-diabetes* just like we need to list *obesity* and *overweight* among the correctable risk factors.

If you take the drugs for Diabetes that boost your insulin production or if you take the very high dose of insulin usually needed in type II diabetes patients who don't follow their diets, you get even higher insulin levels. Again: **High Insulin levels give rise to more arterial plaque**.

As for diet, fruits often will satisfy that urge for sweets without raising the blood sugar as much as candy and the like. If the blood sugar goes up, insulin production goes up. You can't just eat bowl after bowl of fruit. Overdosing on fruit can be as bad as candy for your blood glucose. The insulin production goes up when the sugar is absorbed. In distinction, complex carbohydrates in the form of whole grains and vegetables are absorbed more slowly which stimulates less insulin secretion.

Hyperinsulinism, or insulin resistance is discussed in the chapter at the beginning called "Why have so few patients been told about Insulin Resistance?"

Anyway, that's why I would list Risk Factor #4 as Insulin Resistance rather than obesity, overweight, diabetes, pre-diabetes, and poor diet.

*********************5********************

Smoking is the Big Kahuna of cardiac risk factors. The danger of smoking came out from behind the curtain years ago. That's why I'm not going to spend a lot of time on smoking, it's well known. By the way, smokers tend to get treated more for high blood pressure. Why? It's because smokers usually have a cigarette in the car before coming into the doctor's office. That nicotine assures that your blood pressure reading by the doctor's assistant will be higher than your average for the day. ☼

A Patient With Severe Weight Loss

Perhaps 20 years ago a new patient came to me with the help of one of my long time patients who brought him.

She said, "George lives in our apartment building and I am worried about him. I was hoping you could help him. He has seen all the doctors at XYZ Hospital. They know he has cancer because he has lost so much weight over several months, but all the cancer tests have been negative. They just don't know what to do."

I checked him over. I took a history and could not find anything remarkable or suspicious other than being very thin. I looked at him, I felt him, I probed him, and I listened to his heart and lungs.

A medical student was with me that day. I said to the student: "Whenever you have a patient who is sick and you don't know why, think about ordering blood cultures." That's what I did.

A blood culture detects if the patient has sepsis. The lab tries to grow bacteria from the bloodstream. Normally bacteria in the bloodstream are either not present or are present only very briefly. We know to order this test if the patient has shaking chills and fever. George did not.

The next day I had a call from the lab. His blood specimens were all growing a type of bacteria that is known to be one of the causes of endocarditis. That's an infection of the inside of the heart and the heart valves. It is fatal if not treated.

I hospitalized him and the specialists confirmed the diagnosis of subacute bacterial endocarditis (SBE). His weight loss was not from cancer. It was due to SBE. He was treated for weeks with IV antibiotics. In time, he needed to have his ruined heart valve replaced.

With the subacute type of endocarditis, you're just not that sick at first but you get sicker as time goes on. It sneaks up on you.

Is this a common cause of weight loss? No.

My point is that when all the normal tests fail to show the problem, you need to find a doctor who is a detective and who will think hard and consider possibilities that are "outside of the box."

I'm only a little pleased with my diagnostic skills in this case. I'll tell you why: If you gather enough monkeys and place them in front of typewriters, eventually one will type out a Shakespearean sonnet.

What I mean is that some days practicing medicine you are brilliant and other days you can't see what's in front of you. That's one reason we make the patient come back for follow-ups. If your doctor is not having a sharp day when you are really sick with something, your smart questions may wake up the genius sleeping inside his/ her brain.

So in doctoring, you shouldn't let it go to your head if you are a genius one day and you shouldn't get down if you fail to figure out something the next day.

When you have a medical student with you, it slows you down and gives you more time to think. But I must say I was pretty good at practicing slowly and getting behind schedule without a student's help.

I am retired now. When I was an employed physician I was regularly getting taken to the woodshed about being behind schedule, but I was too stubborn to change. As a patient, I find it reassuring if a doctor keeps me waiting an hour or even two once in a while. My advice: when you go to a doctor, set aside a half-day, bring a book, and chill.

And if you have an idea, share it with your doctor.

About 15 years after George appeared at my office, I was feeling sick for more days than you should blame on a virus.

My doctor checked me and couldn't find anything. He ordered routine blood tests. They were normal. I didn't get better. A few days later, I messaged my doctor and asked him to order some blood cultures, based on that same rule I taught my medical students.

The lab grew the same bacterial species in my blood as my patient George had had. I was admitted for treatment of subacute bacterial endocarditis. I recovered with no heart damage. Early diagnosis is critical for this diagnosis yet the presentation of the illness can be subtle. I am hoping that some day at least one reader of this book is saved by having known about SBE and how hard it is to diagnose and asking their doctor to consider SBE in the workup of their unusual illness.

A Secret Nighttime Swim At Princeton

It seems like you are always at the pool when you are on the swim team. Our practice season started in September and continued through late March. That didn't stop us from sneaking into the Dillon pool during the darkness of night, to swim a little more for fun and adventure. The swimmers had a secret way into the building, a window that looked locked but really wasn't.

One wall above the pool was all windows, so turning on the lights was out of the question. The real adventure was swimming in the dark. A little starlight found its way into the pool but that was it. Swimming in the darkness was tricky. It was hard to tell if you were about to swim into the pool wall. But one advantage was you didn't need a bathing suit. Even if there were spectators, they wouldn't have been able to see a thing, it was that dark.

My friend Tom was a swimmer skilled in the art of sculpture. Tom's ambition was to sculpt a swimmer in the water in a way that had never been done.

I had tinkered with photography in high school. I had taken photos for my school newspaper and yearbook but never did action shots.

In swimming, it's just you and the water. Paddles and fins are not allowed in competition. Goggles? We didn't have them then. Just the swimmer and the water.

Football players could stare at the gridiron. Baseball players could stare at the diamond. What is the image in the mind of a swimmer when he looks at the water? It changes shape so constantly that water is essentially a shapeless thing. The swimmer is surrounded by it, but cannot see it. He cannot feel it to learn its shape. As he touches the water, it moves. But a sculptor could freeze the action and show us something we all experienced every day but could not see.

Different artists had produced castings of swimmers on trophies and medals. They were styled with a kind of formalistic primitivism; they looked like they were created by someone with limited artistic skill and little knowledge of swimming. Sometimes these sculptors simply represented the water as wavy lines.

Tom wanted to bring the sculpture of swimmers to a higher level. He would show how a swimmer really looked in the water and how the water really looked against the swimmer. So we came up with the idea to sneak into the pool at night with a camera and an electronic flash. I would get stop-action photos of him swimming and he would model his sculpture from that.

Why was doing it in the dark so important? We were in college over 50 years ago when superfast camera shutter speeds didn't exist. The best way you could stop the action was with an electronic strobe flash. The camera shutter would open and then close 1/30 of a second later but sometime during that thin slice of time the flash would go off, freezing the action. The strobe only lasted 1/2000 second. The idea was for the flash to be the shutter as it were.

The cameras in that day required a 1/30 second setting for electronic flash synchronization. If you chose 1/500 of a second shutter speed, it might fail to synchronize. The flash might not flash when the camera shutter was open.

We were stuck with a very slow 1/30 second shutter speed. If you shoot with a manual camera, you know that's too slow for action.

To describe the problem a different way: 1/30 second is 33/1000ths or 66/2000ths. During one two-thousandth of a second, the flash would go. During the remaining 65 two-thousandths, the shutter would be open without flash. If we tried to shoot a swimmer with the electronic flash in the daytime with those bright windows at Princeton's Dillon pool, a lot of light would reach the negative in those 65/2000ths sec. The swimmer and the water moved enough during that time that the image wouldn't be sharp on the negative.

Only shooting in the dark could totally freeze the action. That's why we planned our adventure for the dark of night.

We carefully sneaked into Dillon pool. Tom swam back and forth. Looking through the viewfinder I could only see darkness. I could hear him go by better than I could see him. I just shot when I thought he was close. I took many pictures, hoping to get something that would capture the water and the swimmer just right.

After taking the pictures I had to develop the film to see whether we captured what Tom needed.

I recall that night as if it were yesterday.

A few shots did come out well enough. We could see the motionless water's surface as we had never known it. Everything was sharp. Tom used those images to make his sculpture.

With the guidance of Princeton's resident sculptor, Joe Brown, the clay was transformed into bronze.

My friend's sculpture is seen regularly. It has become the swimmer on a piece of wood with an engraved plaque. It is a trophy awarded every year to a member of the swim team who inspires his teammates with his efforts in practice. It is known to Princeton swimmers and divers as the Dermod F. Quinn Memorial Award.

Sneaking into the pool at night was not a legal thing to do. For that reason, we never made this story public. Few people at Princeton today know how that sculpture came into being.

Do Doctors Dislike Caring for People With Addiction?

My first practice was in a fairly rural town. Kennewick was a good-sized city for southeastern Washington State but it was small compared to what I was used to. During my first year of practice, a 30-year-old man came to me.

He told me he was visiting from Canada. He was receiving chemotherapy for a brain tumor but had forgotten his medication. Could I write a prescription for methotrexate, the cancer drug? Oh, and by the way, he also forgot his pain pills.

I wondered. Could he be an addict? But if he were an addict why did he want methotrexate? I decided to give him the benefit of the doubt. I wrote a prescription for two weeks of methotrexate and two weeks of his pain medication. I wrote them on the same prescription and also wrote an order to the pharmacist: "Fill both of these."

Later that day I had a call from the pharmacist. "I had to fill the pain medication for that patient, but he didn't want the methotrexate."

I had been bamboozled at the tender age of 29!

I have learned it's better to use the term "persons with addiction." I like that because it emphasizes the word "person." Do doctors dislike taking care of persons with addiction who are using? In my experience, it is clear that primary care doctors don't enjoy taking care of them unless they are in recovery.

Addiction is just another illness and "using" is just a phase of that disease. Why should doctors dislike caring for patients with addiction who have relapsed?

It is important to explain the difference between habituation and addiction to those who do not know. In addiction, a person repeatedly uses a substance or repeats a behavior despite being increasingly harmed by the activity. Habituation simply means that a person will have a withdrawal reaction if they do not take a substance.

In this essay, I am discussing persons with addiction who are out of control and exhibit drug-seeking behavior. I don't mean those who are in recovery. I don't mean non-addicts who are habituated to stable doses of narcotics for a chronic condition.

Family members who live with people who suffer addiction out of recovery hate what addiction does to them. There is no question they can be difficult to like. Out of control these patients often hurt the people they should love.

Part of the definition of addiction is that the patient in relapse cares more about the substances to which they are addicted than they care about the people who are in their lives.

I'd say most primary care doctors dread having patients who are addicted and not in recovery come into the office as new patients. One problem is they don't have a big sign on their forehead warning everybody that they are seeking drugs. Their stories are very believable. They often put in the request for a narcotic at the end of a long new patient visit.

I knew a doctor who said he solved this problem. He accepted no new patients who were taking pain pills or tranquilizers. No one taking a controlled drug was allowed as his new patient. He solved his problem by leaving all these "tough" patients to the other doctors

But why do doctors get upset? Most ER Doctors or Family Doctors don't have to spend that much time with lapsed addicted patients in the course of a day.

One obvious answer to that question is that people with addiction who are using will lie to get what they want. Lies are confusing to doctors. We rely heavily on what patients tell us. We know some of what the patient says is a lie and some is true. What to believe?

My friend Professor Bill Haning MD, an addiction specialist in Honolulu and President of the American Society of Addiction Medicine, advised me on this chapter. He reminded me these patients are hardly the only ones to confuse their doctors with a dishonest history. Diabetic patients claim they are following their diets. Hypertension patients claim they take their medication every day. I was always pretty good at arithmetic and I must say I did notice a lot of hypertension patients made a 360-day supply, like 90 with three refills, last 420 days or so.

But when seeing that new patient with a painful condition who requests a controlled substance, the doctor thinks, "If I don't diagnose the problem, this patient could get into trouble and then so could I. But if I prescribe controlled substances when not warranted, the state can suspend my license to practice."

So you make a plan. You will diagnose what's going on and treat every aspect of the disease except for the pain. No pain prescription for this patient.

Then the empathy-attack begins. You sense how much pain the patient is suffering. It seems unthinkable not to help. Why not allow just a few pain pills? You prescribe ten. One day later that patient is calling back for more.

You have now started a game called "Can the patient out-fox the doctor?"

You bring back the patient and collect a urine specimen. If it's negative. The patient is selling the pain pills instead of taking them. They sell for $10 to $80 per pill on the street. The doctor wins the game.

Even if the urine test shows the narcotic, you still don't know if the patient took three pills and sold seven.

Are you getting the picture? The patient with addiction can easily be better at this game than the doctor.

In talking with several of my medical students I developed this idea, an explanation of our hangup taking care of these patients. I believe there is a mythology that supports being a doctor. Addicted persons who have relapsed don't fit the pattern of our myth. We don't like that.

Myths are not just a bunch of old tales that go back to ancient Greece and Rome that we are forced to learn in school. Myths are stories that represent patterns of modern life too. Myths establish our culture and our traditions. Myths enlighten the young by teaching lessons learned by the old.

As physicians, we have sacrificed a great deal to get where we are. We gave up personal time and freedom, and we missed many parties and fun times with our friends. We missed time with our spouse and our children. We invested nearly all our energy in our profession, and we lost a ton of sleep along the way to boot. And unless our parents were both well-to-do and generous, to get through school we lost a lot of money in the form of student loans to cover tuition and expenses during our training.

But it's worth it because now, in a sense, we live the "Myth of the Knight in Shining Amour" or for our women doctors let's say "a Moana."

We are privileged to rescue people in distress. What a great job this is! To a great extent, the mental image of this hero/heroine myth applies to nurses too.

As doctors doing this rescuing, as it were, we know some patients are at their worst when they are sick.

In the ancient Greek myth of Perseus and the Gorgon, Princess Andromeda is chained to a sea cliff waiting for the monster to come and eat her. Along comes Perseus with Medusa's head which he must hold in a most awkward fashion behind himself all the while riding Pegasus, the flying horse. As you recall, if anyone looks directly at Medusa they turn to stone. Perseus manages to turn the sea monster to stone without petrifying himself or Andromeda. He has rescued the beautiful princess. I'm telling you: she is not looking her best at that moment. Her hair is wet, she is dirty, she is hungry, she is exhausted, she is stressed out and irritable and it had probably been a while since she'd put on makeup or taken a bath.

When we "rescue" a patient, we get to meet the least appealing version of that person. They may be tired, fearful, angry, worried, distrustful or even unconscious. But we are trained to deal with that: the Knight knows sometimes frogs need to be rescued because "Poof" they can be turned back into a Princess or Prince once the dragon is slain and someone says a few magic words.

If the frog turns back into a Princess or Prince: that's OK. But so often that out-of-recovery patient is a master manipulator who comes across as nice, like a prince or a princess. But then we become super bummed out when it turns out they were really a frog in disguise. We were fooled.

The doctor says, "Did I work this hard for ten years plus to rescue frogs? No!!! Not me!! I'm in the princess-rescuing business. I never learned a myth about the knight who rescued frogs."

So for that patient, your enthusiasm is depleted. When your energy comes back, you try desperately to turn that frog into a prince or princess. Time and time again, despite your best efforts, they remain frogs. I think they only change if and when they make the decision to do so. You try so hard you deplete your energy and that's called being burned out for the day.

After that, if you're not careful, you become permanently bitter and nasty and you might become a frog too. ☼

I think we need a new myth about a kind Knight or heroine whose nobility is enhanced by trying to rescue frog after frog. Even if he/she fails again and again to help the frog into recovery from its frogginess, the noble hero/heroine of this new myth feels a sense of self-worth for having tried.

Let our students model their lives after that myth.

And let's have another new myth about a heroine/hero who time and time again risks the scorn of patients by refusing inappropriately demands to prescribe habit-forming substances for people who don't need them, being cautious even with patients who are not yet addicted or habituated. Praise the nobility of the surgeon who prescribed six pain pills post-op, not 30, with no refills but says "Call me if you need six more in a few days." Praise the family doctor who uses the recommended non-habit-forming antidepressants for patients with anxiety rather than habit-forming tranquilizers.

Understanding a Few Things Can Help You be a Smart Medication Shopper

Many patients are lucky to have the type of insurance that covers medications. Sometimes it's better not to use it every time. ☼

Why wouldn't you use your insurance?

Recently a patient needed a refill of Estrogen Cream. It was $115 with the insurance. It was $55 without the insurance using codes from a GoodRx coupon, available online.

Even with the best pharmacist rooting for you as it were, you may need to say: "Ouch, this one costs more than I expected. Is there another way to buy this medication?"

Some pharmacies have their own discount programs that in many cases will give a much lower price than you pay with your insurance. For some large chains, the pharmacists are not permitted to tell you about GoodRx but they take it if you come in with the coupon (paper or on the phone)

One word of caution: If you anticipate many prescriptions during the year, especially costly ones, paying the higher price may turn out better because you have to consider your deductible. When you buy without using your insurance you don't contribute to your deductible. That's the insurance company's rule. You help them by not using your insurance but they don't help you back.

You will need to do the math. Check the terms of your insurance contract if you don't know your deductable. Compare doing it one way versus the other.

What about calling a different pharmacy? If you go to several pharmacies, they may lose the ability to detect a potential drug interaction. Commonly prescribed medications will be more likely to be the same price. But like other stores, pharmacies may have loss leaders: things that are sold for a very low price to attract you to the store. The Good Rx coupon website will show you the GoodRx price at several local pharmacies when you provide your zip code.

What about generics? Most are just as good as brand-name drugs. They are much less expensive. I have seen generics that had drug recalls. I have seen the same for brand-name drugs. One huge manufacturing plant owned by a Big Pharma company in Puerto Rico was shut for a year or more over quality issues. The FDA actually inspects generic manufacturers overseas, including in China.

Could brand-name drugs be better than generics? Some people buy the argument that if it costs more it must be better.

Here is a story that started in the 1980s. The company that makes Synthroid a brand of levothyroxine, a thyroid replacement identical to human thyroid hormone, a really wonderful drug whether branded or generic, sold their med in umpteen different sizes so the doctor could prescribe the exact dose for each patient. They made tablets of 25, 50, 75, 88, 100, 112, 125, 137, 150, 175, 200 and 300 mcg. They sent around their salespeople to make sure doctors understood how important it was to prescribe their brand and take advantage of all those in-between strengths. I should point out that a different company owns this brand today. The drug has changed hands several times.

In 1987 the company that owned the drug that year, funded a study to show that their Synthroid-branded thyroid replacement product was superior to the generic. A few doctors had a contract to do the research. By 1990 it was apparent that the group that took the Synthroid brand and the other group that took the generic versions had the same outcomes. They all did fine.

Knoll, which had bought the drug in the meantime pulled the funding and prohibited the researchers from publishing their findings. A dispute ensued that lasted six years. The company claimed the study was flawed but had no convincing evidence. The paper was about to be published in 1994 when the University of California at San Francisco, where it was written, refused to release the paper due to fear of a lawsuit from Knoll.

Dr. Sidney Wolfe from the Public Citizen's Health Research Group said "Americans have been bilked out of almost $800 million in extra costs for purchasing the Knoll version of thyroxine because of the suppression of evidence that the other three versions (the generic ones) are just as bioavailable."

In late 1996 the study was finally published. Everybody apologized for putting their own interests above that of the public.

Another way to survive expensive medications is to ask about "compassionate use" programs. Many drug companies have these programs to help their employees feel better about their expensive prices by offering free medication to low-income patients. You apply through your doctor's office. Forms have to be requested and completed and then you wait for the approval.

Another idea is to ask your doctor if there is an older equivalent but different medication that will do the job. The newer drugs don't have generic versions for sale. The older meds are often better. The doctors have been hammered by advertising so much that the new drug pops up in their minds first and sometimes that's the prescription they write. Ask your doctor to think about a lower-cost, older med in the same class of drugs, that might be available as a generic.
☼

One more tricky thing in this business is the opaque dealings of Pharmacy Benefits Managers or PBMs. Often your drug insurance requires going through their contracted PBM to get your meds. You may not have heard the term PBM but you probably have heard the names of the companies: the big ones are CVS Health, Express Scripts, and OptumRx.

Two games they play are called "copay clawbacks" and "spread pricing." The former term means the price paid by the consumer as a copay under the insurance is more than what the PBM pays for the drug. How can your "share" of the cost be more than they paid for it? They tell the patient in the explanation of benefits, "You paid $10 and the insurance paid $10" but the drug actually cost them less than $10. Spread pricing means the amount charged to the insurance company is higher than what the PBM pays to the pharmacy. They make your insurance pay $10 of "the cost" but it really only cost them $5. The difference is retained by the PBM to bloat its profits. This is not the way PBMs are supposed to be making money.

Reference:https://www.healthcaredive.com/news/pbm-practices-consumers-generics-savings-USC/624702/

Here's something even stranger, that I learned a few years ago from a patient: The PBM made a deal with the maker of Adderal XR, a drug used for hyperactive patients. The price was fixed, the PBM got a share of it, but the far less expensive generics were not covered under PBM-managed insurance in any way shape or form.

Theoretically, the job of the PBM is to find the best price for the benefit of the patient and the insurance company. Now, I don't have the insider information, but it was reported in the NY Times that even if the generic cost $10 and the brand name was $90, they would pay for the brand-name but not reimburse that patient who got the generic.

Why not? Because they got a cut on the $90 branded version every time the brand name was filled. And of course,

309

if the patient went out on his own and got the generic, whatever the patient did pay did not go towards the deductible for the year. The PBM covered the more expensive brand-name, hurting the insurance company, as well as the patient, so that they could get their $$$.

Reference:https://www.nytimes.com/2017/08/06/health/prescription-drugs-brand-name-generic.html?smprod=nytcore-ipad&smid=nytcore-ipad-share&_r=0

In summary, don't just accept the price you are told you must pay for your medication. ☼

One last suggestion: let's say you need 300 mg per day of your medication, every day of the year. But 300 mg is not a popular dose so they charge $3 per capsule. You think: what's hidden behind a curtain? Nosey little you asks the pharmacy: "How much are the 100 mg capsules?"

Phamacy: "Oh, let's look it up...they're 25 cents each."

You get your doctor to prescribe three of those per day. Now you are paying 75 cents per day, not $3.00. You save $2.25 each day. That's $821 per year.

You can't fight the PBMs. You need to be a congressman or some other person in power to do that. Be wary of the PBMs.

Mail orders direct from them must be cheaper, right? Wrong: you have to get on line and look it up.

Your Doctor May Not Understand Nutrition☼

According to an article released in 2017 by T.H. Chan at the Harvard School of Public Health, only a fifth of medical schools require a course in nutrition and most schools require less than 25 hours of nutrition education.

https://www.hsph.harvard.edu/news/hsph-in-the-news/doctors-nutrition-education/#:~:text=%E2%80%9CToday%2C%20most%20medical%20schools%20in,in%20nutrition%2C%20it's%20a%20scandal.

I can believe it. I married a dietitian.

I recall it was 1977 and I was in my residency. A doctor put in an order for a special diet. It wasn't me. The doctor told the dietitian it had to be low in carbs because the patient had diabetes, it had to be low in protein because the patient had renal failure and it had to be low in fat because the patient had blood lipid abnormalities. And here's the best part: the diet had to have 3000 calories because the patient was too thin.

This order gave rise to peals of laughter in the dietitians' office. There was one major problem: all foods contain one or more of three ingredients: carbs, proteins, and fats. If you get rid of all three, there's nothing left except water and vitamins.

A Caveman Passes Out

You would think that in a conventional book, a discussion of prehistoric times would be found in the beginning of the book. If you got this far you know this is not a conventional book. Why do people pass out? Nobody knows whether this caveman scenario might be accurate but it is possible that passing out helped early man survive.

Let's pretend you are a prehistoric man or woman and you're being chased by a carnivorous creature with large teeth that can run faster than you and you know it. You are scared out of your mind. It's lucky you are not wearing underwear, which has not been invented. What do you do as you feel the hot breath of the animal on your back as he gets closer and closer?

You do something that you were designed to do, you pass out.

A reflex built into your nervous system causes the blood vessels in the central part of your body to dilate or open up wide. That makes the blood pressure sharply drop. The circulation to your brain decreases and you feel faint and suddenly you pass out. The hungry creature with large teeth approaches your unconscious body lying on the ground.

Nature gave you another survival tool, a terrible body odor. Soap has not yet been invented yet. You have never washed in your life. You're a caveman. You totally stink. You smell like something that died three weeks ago. Not just died, but died and then spoiled.

The creature with the large teeth looks down at your body, sees you are not moving, and notices you smell like something dead and rotten. The creature's survival instinct tells him, "Don't eat rotten food; it can make you sick." So he goes away and a few minutes later you wake up alive and alone. You scurry off to your cave.

Passing out and bad body odor saved your sorry caveman butt.

I don't know whether this story would be believed by a trained paleoanthropologist. But this part is true: we mainly pass out because of stress and fear.

Should young people who pass out get extensive medical testing? Most medical workups are not going to show anything at all in that age-group. ☼ Most of the time, you don't need to do a test for passing out if you are young and healthy.

Passing Out is Common

People frequently pass out, it's something we are programmed to do. Mostly it's a vasovagal reaction. I will explain that term.

There's a part of your brain you cannot command that's working in the background. This section of your brain can control the workings of your body in ways that you cannot voluntarily. Freud called it the unconscious mind.

Often when you pass out, something in the unconscious was emotionally upset over something going on.

The unconscious mind is not logical. What we fear does not need to make sense. A significantly fearful event causes a big physiological discharge from the vagal nerve which causes the vessels inside your trunk to dilate wide open which lowers the blood pressure. Your awareness of these changes due to feeling tingling or lightheadedness further increased the anxiety. That gets the conscious mind involved. The body reacts now to both the unconscious and the conscious mind. You pass out. If you are already sitting on the floor you won't hit anything on the way down. Read between the lines: if you feel faint, don't wait to pass out, get down on the floor now. ☼

According to a study from 2014, the annual number of episodes of passing out is between 18 and 40 per thousand patients. Forty per thousand would be one in 25 people.

That would be up to 4000 episodes of passing out per 100,000 every year.

Most of these spells are in patients between ages 10 and 30. That would be 40,000 per million people or four million per 100 million people. The USA has about 331 million people so that's 13,240,000 cases of passing out per year in the country. Obviously passing out cannot be that dangerous or we wouldn't have many people left.

In fact, heart disease is the most common cause of death and that kills 23% or 635,000 of the 2,750,000 who die in this country every year.

Yet when people pass out, those close to them typically wonder if the episode was a predictor for sudden death, a warning of some type of future disaster. Surely a complete cardiac workup is needed! Or not needed! That depends on your age and underlying medical condition.

The annual incidence of sudden death in the United States, with a population of 331 million, is somewhere between 100,000 and 250,000. If we used 250,000 that would be one in 1200 Americans who die suddenly each year. That is 83 per 100,000. Most of those victims are older.

So let's look at the statistics. Out of 100,000 people, up to 4000 are going to pass out in a year and most of these are young. Sudden death will be suffered by 83 and most of those are old.

Now 4000÷83 is 48 so even without considering age, there will be 48 people passing out for everyone that suddenly dies at a later date. But this math is obviously misleading because most of the people who pass out are younger and most of the people who die suddenly are older.

So if you are younger, maybe you don't need the big workup for passing out unless you have risk factors or there is something else suspicious like a complete lack of warning, like you were fine and the next thing you know you are on the floor checking out the ceiling. That very sudden loss of consciousness suggests a cardiac rhythm disturbance. If you are older your doctor may advise you need the workup. The numbers tell the story.

Most passing out from a vasovagal reaction comes on over a few seconds or longer. If you sense that's happening to you because you feel weird and faint, I repeat, QUICKLY sit down on the ground or lie down to be sure you don't fall.

If you are already flat but still feel faint get someone to lift your legs up higher than your heart. Force your lips into a tight slit and very, very slowly but deeply breathe in and out. I mean each inspiration should take 10 seconds. Each expiration should take ten seconds. I'm sure it would be embarrassing to lie down in a public place like at the mall but it would even be worse if you passed out, broke a bone or your head and they had to call an ambulance.

This way of breathing through a slit in your mouth is called "pursed-lip breathing." You can do this any time you feel anxious. Pursed-lip breathing makes a lot of people feel relaxed. It blocks hyperventilation or rapid breathing. Try it.

THE END

315

INDEX

321

Made in the USA
Monee, IL
23 October 2022

16447336R00188